How small changes
your health and your baby's development

IT
STARTS
WITH THE
BUMP

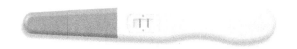

Evidence-based strategies for a
happy and healthy pregnancy

REBECCA FETT
—AUTHOR OF IT STARTS WITH THE EGG

FRANKLIN
FOX

It Starts with the Bump

ISBN-13 (print): 979-8-9886751-8-1
ISBN-13 (ebook): 979-8-9886751-9-8

Contents

Introduction

THE MOMENT THOSE two lines appear, the world shifts, heralding the start of a new chapter. The goal of this book is to offer a road map to what comes next, so you can rest assured that you're on the right path without having to research every question, trawl through a sea of conflicting data, or wonder if you may be missing something important.

One of the challenges in making the best health decisions during pregnancy is the glacial pace at which official recommendations are updated based on new scientific research. After a breakthrough, it can often take a decade or longer for health professionals to implement practical changes. I hope to reduce that gap by sharing some of the most important new findings, so you can take a proactive role in your pregnancy, advocate for yourself, and make informed decisions every step of the way.

As a science writer, I've spent much of the past decade sharing the latest medical research findings and translating complex science into practical guidance. This is something I care deeply about because I've seen firsthand just how much impact new scientific research can have on people's lives, including my own.

As you may know from reading my first book, *It Starts with the Egg*, I was told in my twenties that I had poor ovarian function and very little chance of conceiving, even with IVF. I found it hard to accept that everything was out of my hands and decided to put my training in molecular biology and biochemistry to work. I spent months delving into the scientific research and found a plethora of new discoveries that had not yet filtered down into mainstream medical practice. I then translated those discoveries into a plan of action to improve my egg quality and ovarian function, using supplements, dietary changes, and minimizing exposure to certain toxins. Approaching the problem from a scientific angle, I focused on the steps that should make the most difference according to the underlying chemistry and biology.

This turned out to be the right approach and within just a few months, I saw a dramatic improvement. I went from worrying whether any eggs could be retrieved to getting a large number of good-quality embryos from a single IVF cycle, including two embryos that eventually became my baby boys.

Knowing that vital information in the scientific literature was not being shared with those who needed it, I felt compelled to go further. I analyzed every relevant study I could find and developed a systematic approach to help others struggling with infertility or recurrent miscarriage. The resulting book took on a life of its own. Now in its third edition, *It Starts with the Egg* is recommended by a wide array of IVF clinics and fertility specialists. On a daily basis, I hear from women who have followed the strategies in that book and are finally pregnant after years of infertility and multiple failed

IVF cycles, or who have finally reached a major milestone in their pregnancy after multiple losses.

For those who are newly pregnant after reading my earlier book, the natural question is: what next? How can we take the same approach of proactively learning from the latest scientific research and apply it to pregnancy in order to optimize maternal health, reduce the likelihood of complications, and nurture a baby's growth and development? That's the subject of this book. It's intended not just for those who are pregnant after a difficult path, but anyone who simply wants to have the healthiest pregnancy possible, based on the most up-to-date information.

You'll learn ways to manage common pregnancy symptoms, prepare your body for labor and delivery, and nourish your baby's developing brain. We'll also cover strategies to optimize the health of the placenta—a topic that takes on greater importance if you are in your late 30s or early 40s, conceived through IVF, or have certain medical conditions. As you'll learn in the chapters to come, new research has shown that the placenta may function slightly differently in these situations, necessitating a little more care and attention.

If you fall into this category, your doctor will likely perform additional monitoring during the third trimester and may recommend earlier induction. Your pregnancy may be labeled "high risk" even if the only relevant factor is your age or having conceived by IVF.

In reality, the chance of any complication remains quite low, so a more appropriate label might be "low-ish risk," but it is still worth understanding why your pregnancy might warrant closer monitoring and how the risks of complications can be reduced even further.

Fortunately, the latest scientific research now provides clear guidance on that topic. Studies have shown that it's possible to significantly reduce the chance of developing high blood pressure and various other complications related to the placenta. We can do so by supporting blood flow and reducing inflammation during the first half of pregnancy, when the all-important connection between the mother's and baby's blood supply is forming. Later in pregnancy, taking aspirin and certain supplements can also help prevent complications. Standard medical advice rarely covers this important topic because the focus is typically on diagnosis and treatment rather than prevention. When it comes to the health of the placenta, a better approach is to act early to reduce the odds of a problem ever occurring.

Our goal goes far beyond that, however. The strategies covered in this book aim to support your overall health throughout pregnancy—not only to reduce the chance of complications but also to ease pregnancy symptoms, support your baby's growth, and ensure an easier postpartum recovery.

Although the main focus is supporting your physical health, looking after your mental and emotional health is just as important. This book gives you some practical strategies for doing so, to help ease some of the worry and nervousness that are so common in early pregnancy.

Over the past ten years of supporting readers of *It Starts with the Egg*, I've noticed a near-universal feeling among those who are pregnant after a difficult path: they want to do everything possible to nurture this hard-won pregnancy, but they also wish they could let go of some of the anxiety and experience a little more joy and excitement.

Some degree of self-protective worry is perfectly valid and justified, especially if you've faced years of heartbreak to get here. Even so, you also deserve to enjoy this time. I want to help you navigate this balancing act by providing evidence-based tools for managing anxiety during times of uncertainty. You'll learn how to pull yourself out of stress mode and shift into a state of calm. Instead of being at the mercy of every anxious or negative thought that comes along, you'll be able to reassure yourself that the odds are on your side and you're doing the best for your baby. Then you can go through your pregnancy with less worry and more peace.

Before delving into the specific practical steps you can take to optimize both your mental and physical health, it's worth noting that you don't need to put everything mentioned in this book into practice. You can choose which topics to focus on and which to set aside. Your body is designed to nurture and deliver a healthy baby—it knows what to do. We're simply providing a little extra help where we can.

If you're short on time or feeling overwhelmed, you can start with the bullet-point summaries at the end of each chapter, then refer back to the more detailed guidance if and when you need it. This is your pregnancy, and you get to choose your own adventure.

Finding Your Way

The first chapters focus on optimizing your supplement routine, with guidance on choosing the best prenatal, the optimal doses of vitamin D and iron, and determining which other supplements you may need to start or stop.

Although it's usually best to take a minimalist approach to supplements during pregnancy, several supplements can help overcome deficiencies in our modern diets. As discussed in Chapters 1–3, the most useful supplements to add beyond a prenatal include choline, vitamin D, and omega-3 fatty acids. These nutrients not only support your own health during pregnancy but also help support your baby's development.

Certain supplements may also be worth adding if you have any risk factors for gestational diabetes, preeclampsia, or other complications. Chapter 4 covers the pros and cons of low-dose aspirin for preventing preeclampsia and complications related to the placenta. Chapter 5 explains the value of myo-inositol for those with higher odds of developing gestational diabetes due to age, BMI, or medical history.

The other side of the equation is deciding which supplements to stop taking. If you're coming into pregnancy after a struggle with infertility or miscarriage, you may have been taking a fairly comprehensive supplement regime that needs to be pared back. Generally, most fertility and miscarriage supplements should be discontinued when you get a positive pregnancy test. The exceptions may be coenzyme Q10 (CoQ10) and N-acetylcysteine (NAC), which may be helpful during the first trimester if you have a history of recurrent miscarriage, as Chapter 6 explains. This chapter also provides guidance on the controversies over progesterone treatment to prevent miscarriage. A complete summary of the supplements to consider at each stage of pregnancy can be found in the appendix at the end of the book.

Chapters 7 and 8 cover the most important lab tests that may help you spot issues early, such as anemia and low thyroid function. Chapter 9 covers noninvasive prenatal testing, explaining the preferred timing and why some results are typically reliable whereas others should be viewed with skepticism.

Once you have your supplements sorted and early lab tests completed, you may find yourself in a holding pattern, waiting for more reassurance that your pregnancy is going well. During this stage, it can help to learn some tools for managing moments of anxiety and feeling more joy in challenging times. That's the subject of Chapter 10, which shares strategies for diffusing worry and coping with uncertainty using approaches developed by leading psychologists and backed by years of research.

Chapters 11 through 13 share expert advice on managing pregnancy nausea and untangling the controversies over alcohol, caffeine, pregnancy-safe foods, and minimizing exposure to toxins. Chapter 14 focuses on how to safely build core strength and stability for an easier pregnancy and delivery.

Subsequent chapters help you make informed decisions on topics such as pregnancy vaccines, induction, pain relief during labor, and preparing for a C-section. The final chapters focus on caring for your newborn, including troubleshooting breastfeeding, choosing the best formula, and other ways to make the early months as happy and healthy as possible for both you and your baby.

PART 1

Supplements for a Healthy Pregnancy

Chapter 1

Choosing the Best Prenatal Supplement

O NE OF THE most important steps in the early weeks of pregnancy is choosing a good-quality prenatal multivitamin. The right prenatal provides a range of vitamins and minerals needed for a healthy pregnancy, including vitamin A, B vitamins, choline, and iron.

In a perfect world, we'd get all these nutrients from our food, but that's become challenging in modern times. With rising costs and limited time to prepare meals from scratch, it can be difficult to prioritize the most nutrient-dense whole foods. The foods that nourished our ancestors, such as fish, eggs, meat, fruit, vegetables, and legumes, are now often replaced with refined grains and processed foods. Compounding the problem is the fact that fruits and vegetables may be lower in vitamins and minerals than in years past, due to depleted soils and the loss of vitamins before produce reaches store shelves.

Supplements can't solve this problem entirely, but they can make up for some of the shortfall.

What to Look for in a Prenatal

A good-quality prenatal will contain the active or natural form of certain vitamins, instead of synthetic forms. As the next section explains, these natural forms are more readily absorbed and converted into the forms used by our cells. It's also preferable to select a brand that provides the full spectrum of essential vitamins and minerals, including lesser-known B vitamins such as thiamin and riboflavin. As you'll learn later in this chapter, choline is another key nutrient for a healthy pregnancy. Prenatals are often lacking in choline so it may need to be added on as a standalone supplement.

1. Methylfolate

One of the main factors to consider when choosing a prenatal supplement is the form of folate. Over the past decade, many higher-end supplement companies have switched over from synthetic folic acid to the natural form, methylfolate. This switch occurred in response to data suggesting that individuals with certain genetic variants linked to folate metabolism may have higher rates of miscarriage and neural tube defects. By providing folate in the active form, these genetic variations can be circumvented, improving the odds of having a healthy pregnancy.

Balanced against this consideration is the fact that most official guidelines recommend synthetic folic acid. That is because the large clinical trials demonstrating a reduction in neural tube defects only studied that form. In the absence of similar trials using methylfolate, the more conservative approach is to recommend the standard supplement form.

There is good reason to believe that methylfolate would have the same benefits, however, given the underlying science. Folic acid must be converted to natural forms, such as methylfolate, before it is used by our cells. In addition, what matters for preventing neural tube defects is the level of folate in the blood and most of this is methylfolate.[1] Taking methylfolate is also more effective at raising blood folate levels.[2] One would expect from all this data that methylfolate should be just as effective, if not better, at preventing neural tube defects. In any case, the point becomes moot at around 30 days after conception, when the neural tube closes. After that time, folate is taken for other reasons and methylfolate may have other advantages.

As one example, natural folate appears to have a more positive impact on infant brain development during pregnancy. Researchers in Spain found that compared to supplementing with folic acid, a higher intake of natural folate during pregnancy was associated with significantly higher scores in verbal memory and several other key measures of cognitive function when children reached age four or five.[3]

Folate also plays an important role in preventing anemia since it's needed to produce new red blood cells. Taking methylfolate plus additional B12 can prevent pregnancy-related anemia much more effectively than a standard prenatal containing folic acid.[4] As discussed in Chapter 8, preventing anemia benefits you and your baby in a variety of ways, including fewer infections and improved cognitive function.

For all these reasons, it's important to ensure an adequate intake of folate, preferably in the form of methylfolate. Labeling can be confusing due to government regulation, but the specific form of folate is usually identified in brackets in the ingredients list. Methylfolate may be referred to by that name or as 5-methyltetrahydrofolate. The recommended dose is 400–800 mcg per day. If you're unable to find a prenatal containing methylfolate, one option is to take a conventional multivitamin and add a standalone methylfolate supplement of 400 mcg per day.

For a small number of individuals, supplementing with methylfolate may cause mild anxiety or muscle aches. These side effects can be the result of genetic variants or a deficiency in other B vitamins, particularly B12. If you find that methylfolate bothers you, one option is to take a standard multivitamin containing 400 mcg of folic acid, along with a 400-mcg supplement of folinic acid—another natural type of folate that's usually well tolerated and easily converted to active forms. You could also choose a prenatal that contains folinic acid, such as Seeking Health's methyl-free prenatal.

If you live in a country with few supplement options, or if budget is a factor, the best option may be to take a standard multivitamin and focus on consuming more foods rich in natural folate, such as broccoli, cauliflower, leafy greens, legumes, and strawberries. These foods include a combination of methylfolate and other forms of natural folate that are readily converted and used by cells throughout the body.

2. The Full Spectrum of B Vitamins

Although folate gets most of the attention, other B vitamins play a similar role and are likely just as helpful. We know, for instance, that folate depends on these other B vitamins to have its full biological effects. This is particularly true for B6, B12, thiamin, and riboflavin, all of which work together with folate for many biological processes. These B vitamins are likely just as important as folate for preventing neural tube defects.

Vitamins B6, B12, riboflavin, and thiamin are also important because they participate in hundreds of other biological processes, including the production of new blood cells and neurotransmitters, as well as supporting liver function and energy metabolism. For that reason, some of the heavily marketed prenatals that contain folate but neglect the other B vitamins are not the best choice.

The amount of each B vitamin can vary between prenatal brands, but a wide range of doses is acceptable. The goal is to choose a brand that provides somewhere between 100% and 600% of the recommended daily intake for the major B vitamins, including thiamin, riboflavin, B6, biotin, and pantothenic acid. The dosage of B12 is typically much higher, as discussed later in this chapter.

The form of some of these other B vitamins may also matter for some people. Just as folate exists in a standard supplement form and a more biologically active form, the same is true for other B vitamins. As one example, most prenatals contain vitamin B6 as pyridoxine. Before it can participate in the hundreds of reactions in our bodies that require B6, pyridoxine must be converted into the biologically active form, pyridoxal-5-phosphate (P5P). Most people can perform this conversion well, so it isn't a major issue, but the pyridoxine form sometimes causes side effects, such as nausea or headaches. If you suspect you're reacting poorly to your prenatal, you could try a brand that has B6 in the form of P5P, such as Thorne or Designs for Health.

Choosing a prenatal that contains active P5P is a higher priority if you have symptoms of B6 deficiency, such as cracked lips, low mood or anxiety, or frequent infections. Anecdotally, some people with these symptoms show a greater improvement when supplementing with B6 in the active form, particularly if the issue is anxiety or depression. This is likely due to the significant role P5P plays in the production of feel-good neurotransmitters such as serotonin and dopamine.

Vitamin B6 at higher doses is also the first-line treatment for morning sickness (often in combination with the antihistamine doxylamine, which is found in Unisom sleep aids). The usual recommendation is to take 10–25 milligrams of B6, three times a day, plus 10– 20 milligrams of doxylamine at bedtime. Doing so provides the same active ingredients as the prescription medication Diclegis, which is FDA-approved to treat pregnancy nausea. If following this regimen doesn't help enough or causes side effects, you could try a B6 supplement in the form of P5P at the same dose.

Another B vitamin that exists in different supplement forms is riboflavin. Although most brands contain the standard form, some instead contain the more biologically active form known as riboflavin-5-phosphate (R5P). This form may be helpful if you have signs of a riboflavin deficiency. Symptoms include cracked lips or corners of the mouth, a chronic sore throat, or red, itchy eyes.

The final B vitamin important in a prenatal is B12. Similar to folate, B12 plays a role in detoxification and producing new red blood cells. The amount of B12 in a quality prenatal can often seem very high, but that's necessary since B12 is poorly absorbed from oral supplements. The average person absorbs around 1–2% of a supplement dose, so a prenatal labeled as providing 2,000% of the recommended daily intake likely provides at most 40% of your daily B12 needs.

Many prenatals include a much smaller amount, but this is usually only a problem if you are vegan or vegetarian, or if you have a condition that impairs absorption or increases the demand for B12. Conditions associated with low B12 include MTHFR gene variations, autoimmune conditions, celiac disease and other intestinal problems, and taking metformin or medications for acid reflux. If you have any of these conditions or are anemic, testing your B12 levels might be advisable to determine if you have a deficiency.

When assessing your B12 intake, relying solely on total serum B12 measurements may not provide enough information. Even if that level is high, your cells may not be able to access or process B12 effectively. A better approach is to test for active B12, known as Holo-Tc, which should have a value over 60 pmol/L. A more expensive—but even more accurate—test for B12 deficiency measures a metabolite called methylmalonic acid (MMA), which accumulates when B12 is in short supply. Ideally, MMA should be less than 270 nmol/L. A higher level suggests you may need more B12.

3. Vitamin A for Growth and Immunity

Vitamin A regulates the function of more than five hundred genes in the body. During pregnancy, it supports immune function, embryo growth, and the development of your baby's bones, heart, and nervous system. It also lowers the odds of preterm birth and anemia.[5] In addition, this vitamin boosts the immune system, reducing the odds of infection for both mother and baby.[6] One recent study found that babies born with higher vitamin A levels are much less likely to develop a serious infection in their first weeks.[7]

Despite this clear data, many doctors cause unnecessary confusion by advising their pregnant patients to avoid foods and supplements that contain vitamin A. This is particularly common in Britain, where flawed NHS guidelines warn against the "preformed" versions of vitamin A, such as retinyl palmitate and the natural vitamin A found in cod liver oil. Those guidelines advise that only the beta-carotene form is safe during pregnancy.

This concern is not supported by the data. It is based on a single study published more than thirty years ago. The study reported a slight increase in birth defects in women consuming extremely high levels of preformed vitamin A during early pregnancy.[8] Importantly, the dose associated with this increased risk of birth defects was more than 10,000 IU per day from supplements or a total of 15,000 IU per day from diet and supplements combined. These doses are vastly higher than the amount found in modern prenatal supplements, which typically contain less than 3,000 IU.

In Britain and some other countries, the concern over extremely high doses of vitamin A was somehow translated into a blanket advisory against supplementing with preformed vitamin A altogether. This advice ignores the many important roles this vitamin plays during pregnancy and the fact that it is more readily absorbed than its precursor, beta-carotene.

Also ignored is an important point in the 1995 study regarding timing. Specifically, the increase in birth defects was seen only when the high doses of vitamin A were taken during the first seven weeks of pregnancy. After that point, the relevant structures of the embryo have already formed, so birth defects linked to excess vitamin A no longer pose a concern.

In the decades since that initial study, no further research has found evidence of harm from reasonable doses of preformed vitamin A during pregnancy. On the contrary, the most recent studies emphasize the importance of vitamin A for supporting your baby's growth and preventing infection.[9]

In the U.S., the official guidance is more in line with this positive data. The FDA recommends a daily intake of 1,300–2,400 mcg Retinol Activity Equivalents (RAE) per day during pregnancy, which is equivalent to 8,000 IU. Your prenatal likely contains much less, and it may be in the form of beta-carotene, which is quite difficult for the body to absorb and use.[10] Yet this isn't a major problem because most people get enough preformed vitamin A from food. The best food sources of vitamin A are butter, meat, eggs, and full-fat dairy, particularly grass-fed versions. These foods provide vitamin A as retinols, which are readily absorbed and converted into the forms of vitamin A your body uses.

If you are vegan, it can be more challenging to get enough vitamin A from food because plant sources only provide beta-carotene. To compensate for the difficulty of absorbing and converting this form into active vitamin A, a higher intake is needed. The best sources of beta-carotene are bright orange vegetables such as sweet potato, carrots, pumpkin, and winter squash. Broccoli and kale are also good sources. Cooking vegetables well and adding a fat such as olive oil boosts the absorption of beta-carotene.

If you're concerned about a vitamin A deficiency because you have a limited diet, or if you typically struggle with frequent infections or anemia, you may want to have your serum retinol level tested. According to the World Health Organization, serum retinol should be above 0.70 µmol/L during pregnancy.[11] If you need to supplement, a reasonable dose is a 10,000 IU capsule, twice per week, ideally in the form of preformed vitamin A from natural sources. Addressing a deficiency is particularly helpful if you have anemia because vitamin A is needed for the absorption and processing of iron.[12]

4. Choline for Brain Building

Choline is another essential nutrient that provides a range of benefits during pregnancy. They include supporting liver function, preventing neural tube defects, and helping your baby produce new brain cells.[13] Choline plays such an important role in brain development during pregnancy that the benefits of supplementing can be seen in children's brain function many years later.[14] As one example, researchers at the Harvard School of Public Health found that higher choline intake during the first and second trimesters was associated with significantly better visual memory in seven-year-olds.[15]

Because a growing baby is constantly producing so many new cells, including billions of brain cells that each require choline, the demand for this essential nutrient is much higher during pregnancy. Official guidelines typically call for an intake of at least 450 milligrams per day during early pregnancy and at least 550 milligrams per day in the second and third trimesters.

Eggs are by far the best source of this nutrient, with three egg yolks providing 450 milligrams of choline. Eating eggs more often also boosts your intake of many other nutrients, including vitamins A and B12, while providing a good source of protein and keeping blood sugar levels steady. Eating eggs regularly can be a challenge when nausea is at its peak, but fortunately the critical period for choline intake is the second half of pregnancy, when nausea has often subsided.

Choline is also found in other animal foods and, to a lesser extent, some plant foods. However, obtaining enough from these sources can be difficult. After eggs, the foods highest in choline are soybeans, chicken, and beef, but you'd need to consume two cups of soybeans or twelve ounces of chicken or beef every day to meet the recommended intake. As a result, deficiencies are quite common.[16]

To address this gap, the American Medical Association passed a unanimous resolution advocating for greater amounts of choline in prenatals. Many manufacturers have heeded this call and increased the amount to 250 milligrams or more. The optimal supplement dose is likely higher, at around 350 milligrams per day, but this is challenging to fit into a prenatal without increasing the number of capsules. If your prenatal contains at least 250 milligrams, you should be able to make up the shortfall through food, especially if you're able to eat eggs.

If your prenatal has less, the solution is to either eat eggs every day or add a separate choline supplement. Standalone choline supplements often provide 350 milligrams per capsule, which is a good dose for most people. For vegans, a higher-dose supplement, such as 500 milligrams per day, may be needed.

Some studies have indicated that an even higher intake of choline may provide greater benefits to infant brain development.[17] As one example, a randomized study comparing 480 milligrams to 930 milligrams of choline per day in the third trimester found that the higher dose was associated with improved attention spans later in childhood.[18] It is a personal decision whether to opt for this higher intake, but the evidence is not yet strong enough to change the general recommendations.

Research has also suggested that the type of choline found in egg yolks is better absorbed and more effective than the standard supplement form, known as choline bitartrate.[19] There may be some truth to this, but the differences are relatively minor. Choline bitartrate is still a good option; what matters most is simply getting enough choline, regardless of the form.

Other types of choline found in supplements, such as phosphatidylcholine and GPC choline, may also be slightly better than choline bitartrate, but these forms usually require many capsules to achieve the recommended dose. To reach 350 milligrams of choline from phosphatidylcholine, you'd need to take approximately 2,500 milligrams, which is typically six capsules.

In recent years, there has been some controversy over whether taking choline supplements or eating more eggs may increase a metabolite known as TMAO (trimethylamine N-oxide), which has been suspected to increase blood clotting and cardiovascular issues.[20] Concerns over TMAO appear to be unfounded, however, because eating eggs or taking choline supplements only causes a brief rise in this compound, which does not appear to pose any problem.[21] It is quickly excreted and levels return to the same baseline, regardless of choline intake.[22] There is a much greater temporary rise in TMAO after eating fish, and this is not associated with any negative cardiovascular effects.

The bottom line is that choline is part of our natural biology, and it plays an important role in pregnancy. Getting enough is crucial for your baby's brain development and overall well-being, and you can choose whichever form is most convenient.

As discussed in more detail in Chapter 18, continuing your choline supplement when breastfeeding may have further benefits. Choline is a key component of breast milk, although the concentration varies depending on the mother's intake. To optimize your baby's nutrition, the recommended intake is 550 milligrams per day while nursing. To reach that level, you can likely continue the same regime from pregnancy, whether by relying on a supplement or eating eggs most days (or a combination of the two).

Troubleshooting Supplement Side Effects

If you struggle with significant nausea or headaches and taking your prenatal seems to make matters worse, it can be tempting to stop taking supplements altogether. Nausea usually peaks around weeks 6 to 14, and it is generally not a problem to take a break from supplements during this time if you need to. But you may also be able to find a solution that works.

One of the most likely culprits is zinc, which commonly causes nausea when taken on an empty stomach. Taking your prenatal after a meal can sometimes solve this problem. You may also feel better with a prenatal that contains zinc in the form of zinc bisglycinate, which is gentler on the stomach than standard forms.

If your prenatal is still contributing to nausea, or if you suspect it's causing headaches, the issue may be the dose or form of B vitamins. As mentioned earlier, a prenatal with B6 in the active form (as P5P) may be less likely to bother you and may even reduce nausea. You could also try switching to a children's multivitamin or a prenatal with a lower dose of B vitamins.

Another potential troublemaker is iron. Standard forms of iron, such as ferrous sulfate, can sometimes cause significant nausea, vomiting, or constipation. This situation is much less likely to occur with a better form of iron, such as iron bisglycinate chelate. If a prenatal containing that form is hard to find, you can instead take an iron-free multivitamin or a B-complex and add iron bisglycinate separately if needed. As covered in more detail in Chapter 8, many women only need to supplement with additional iron in the second and third trimesters, when nausea has often passed.

Key Points

- A good-quality prenatal should provide 400–800 micrograms of folate, preferably as methylfolate rather than synthetic folic acid.

- It should also include roughly 100%–600% of the recommended daily intake for the other major B vitamins.

- Vitamin A in the form of retinyl palmitate is important during pregnancy for preventing anemia and supporting growth and immunity. If your prenatal includes vitamin A only in the form of beta-carotene, it's helpful to emphasize food sources of preformed vitamin A, such as grass-fed butter.

- Choline plays many important roles during pregnancy, but many prenatals don't contain enough. To reach the recommended daily intake, you'll likely need to eat eggs on most days or take a separate choline supplement. The preferred dose is around 350 milligrams, but this is only a ballpark figure; you can take a higher or lower dose.

- If your prenatal is making nausea worse, you may have better luck with a low-dose children's multivitamin or a brand with better forms of zinc, B vitamins, and iron.

- For recommended supplement brands, see itstartswiththebump.com/supplements

Chapter 2

Preventing Preterm Birth with Omega-3s

THE FAROE ISLANDS are a series of remote and rocky islands in the North Atlantic with a population of just 50,000. These islands may sound like an unlikely place for scientific breakthroughs, yet they have two unique characteristics. The women there eat a lot of fish. They also have one of the lowest rates of preterm birth in the world. Dr. Sjurdur Olsen, then a medical researcher on the islands, was the first to suggest there may be a link between the two. He published a 1986 paper hypothesizing that high intake of omega-3 fats from fish could lower the risk of preterm birth.[1]

It has taken decades to prove that Dr. Olsen was right, but we now have a convincing body of evidence that omega-3 fats do indeed prevent preterm birth. Numerous randomized controlled studies have demonstrated that increasing omega-3 fats during pregnancy lowers the risk of delivering before 34 weeks by more than 40%.[2]

Consuming more omega-3 fats is likely to be even more beneficial for women who would otherwise be very deficient. We know this from Dr. Olsen's latest research, which is still focused on the question of omega-3 fats and preterm birth, thirty years after his initial discovery. Most recently, he and his colleagues directly measured the levels of omega-3 fats in women's blood during the first and second trimesters of pregnancy. They found that women with very low omega-3 fats were ten times more likely to deliver prematurely.[3]

This is a key point for women already facing slightly higher odds of delivering early because of risk factors such as age, conception by IVF, high BMI, or a short interval between pregnancies. Instead of layering on another risk factor in the form of omega-3 deficiency, we can significantly improve the odds of carrying to term. According to Philippa Middleton, an Associate Professor of Pediatrics and Reproductive Health in Australia: "There are not many options for preventing premature birth, so these new findings are very important for pregnant women, babies, and the health professionals who care for them."[4]

It has taken far too long for the link between omega-3 fats and preterm birth to come to light—and the information is still not being shared widely enough. Even so, many pregnant women are already taking a step in the right direction by supplementing with DHA (docosahexaenoic acid), which is often included in prenatal multivitamins.

DHA is one of the main omega-3 fats found in fish and is commonly recommended during pregnancy to support brain growth. Because DHA is used as a building block to produce new brain cells, a growing baby needs a steady supply of it throughout pregnancy. This demand increases significantly during the third trimester, when the brain accumulates DHA at an astonishing rate. Babies accumulate more DHA over these three months than in the 18 months after they are born.[5]

Supplementing with DHA during pregnancy is thought to support this important brain-building process, with the hope of improving a baby's cognitive development.[6] The data on this point is somewhat inconsistent, but several studies have found that supplementing with DHA during pregnancy improves brain function even many years later in childhood.[7] Higher omega-3 intake during pregnancy may also reduce the odds of a child later developing food allergies and asthma.[8]

A further potential benefit is improved blood sugar control in women with gestational diabetes.[9] The improvements in glucose and insulin levels after supplementing with omega-3 fatty acids are often subtle, but the downstream benefits for the baby can be impressive. In one double-blind study of women with gestational diabetes who were given 1,000 milligrams of omega-3 fatty acids for six weeks, less than 8% of babies developed jaundice and needed to stay in the hospital for treatment, compared to 33% in the placebo group.[10]

To achieve all these benefits, and particularly to reduce the risk of preterm birth, taking a prenatal containing a small amount of DHA is probably not sufficient.

The prenatals that include DHA typically provide only 50–200 milligrams, which is far short of the amount needed to reduce the odds of preterm birth.[11] As noted by Dr. Middleton, who analyzed all the studies in this area, "Our review found the optimum dose was a daily supplement containing between

500 and 1,000 milligrams of long-chain omega-3 fats (containing at least 500 milligrams of DHA)."[12]

The other problem with relying on a prenatal to provide DHA is that prenatals typically don't include the other important omega-3 fat, EPA (eicosapentaenoic acid). DHA and EPA work in slightly different ways to reduce the inflammatory molecules that can compromise the health of the placenta and contribute to premature labor. Taking both forms is therefore likely to give the maximum benefit.

One way to ensure you're getting enough omega-3 fatty acids is to add a fish oil supplement that is concentrated enough to provide at least 500 milligrams of DHA and 200 milligrams of EPA in one or two capsules. The precise ratio between the two is not critical. What matters is getting enough DHA along with at least some EPA.

In recent years, concerns have been raised over whether these delicate oils become rancid or oxidized when in supplement form, thus rendering them ineffective. The extent to which this occurs largely depends on the freshness of the bottle and the manufacturer's quality-control processes. Apart from checking that your bottle has at least six months before the expiration date, it helps to choose a brand that prevents oxygen exposure during manufacturing. Nordic Naturals, for instance, manufactures their fish oils in a nitrogen environment to prevent oxidation.

Certification from a third-party testing organization such as IFOS (International Fish Oil Standards) is another good indicator. By choosing an omega-3 supplement labeled as IFOS-certified, you can rest assured that batches are regularly tested to ensure low levels of oxidization.

For current brand recommendations, see itstartswiththe-bump.com/supplements.

Vegetarians and vegans should look for an omega-3 supplement made from algae oil, such as Nordic Naturals Algae Omega. The human body can produce a very small amount of DHA from other plant-based omega-3 fats, including flaxseed oil, but not nearly enough to meet a growing baby's needs. Studies have confirmed that many plant-based omega-3 supplements and oils don't significantly increase DHA levels in pregnant women. Algae-based supplements are much more effective.[13]

As with any supplement, especially when you're pregnant, check with your doctor before adding omega-3 to your regime. One common question is whether fish oil may increase bleeding risk in people taking blood-thinning medication such as Lovenox or Clexane. Because very little evidence exists to support this concern, many obstetricians still recommend fish oil supplements to patients who are on blood-thinning medications, but it's something to discuss with your doctor.[14]

If you've previously delivered early, whether due to immune problems or an unknown cause, consider taking an even higher dose of fish oil. In a study of high-risk women who previously delivered early, supplementing with 2,700 milligrams of combined EPA and DHA per day reduced the chance of another preterm birth by one-third.[15]

When to Stop Omega-3

The flipside of the extraordinary ability of omega-3 fats to prevent preterm birth is that taking high doses toward the end of pregnancy may slightly increase the odds of continuing past your due date or needing an induction.[16]

The data on this is not entirely clear, and any effect is likely quite small, but it's probably best to stop taking omega-3 supplements once you reach 36 weeks to allow for the natural inflammation and hormone production needed to trigger labor. By this time, your baby will have already built up a good supply of DHA.

If you plan to breastfeed, you might consider restarting your omega-3 supplement at some point after you deliver. This is optional and likely much less important than getting adequate DHA during pregnancy, but it significantly increases the omega-3 content of breast milk. We also know that babies need a continuing source of DHA to support brain development and regulate their immune systems. A recent study found that supplementing with omega-3 fats during both pregnancy and breastfeeding reduces the chance of a child developing a peanut allergy by almost 40%.[17]

Getting Omega-3s Directly from Fish

It's possible to get all the omega-3 fats that you and your baby need just by eating cold-water fish such as salmon and sardines. You would need to eat two or three standard-size servings each week of the fish with the highest omega-3 levels. These include:

- salmon
- sardines
- Atlantic mackerel
- herring

Most other types of fish and seafood are too low in omega-3 fats to help you reach the target levels. To obtain sufficient DHA from tuna, shrimp, or flaky white fish such as cod, you would need to eat at least 30 ounces per week, or one serving every day. In the case of tuna, this would put you over the safe level of mercury.

It is widely recognized that excessive mercury during pregnancy can compromise the baby's developing brain.[18] But this shouldn't discourage you from eating fish during pregnancy. It just means that it's important to choose varieties that are lower in mercury. According to the FDA's chief scientist, "the latest science strongly indicates that eating 8 to 12 ounces per week of a variety of fish lower in mercury during pregnancy benefits fetal growth and development."[19] Salmon and sardines are among the best choices because both are very low in mercury and high in beneficial omega-3 fats. A chart comparing the mercury and omega-3 content of other common fish can be found at itstartswiththebump.com/mercury.

Sushi and Smoked Salmon

Pregnant women have long been told to avoid eating raw and smoked fish. The concern is that these foods may harbor parasites or bacteria that could cause food poisoning. Although food poisoning is a greater concern during pregnancy, current recommendations are somewhat overcautious when it comes to sushi.

In the United States, the FDA advises that raw fish is not safe to eat while pregnant because it may contain parasites or bacteria, including salmonella. Yet the risk from consuming sushi-grade raw fish is actually very low, particularly if the fish was previously frozen. The British National Health Service has in fact updated its guidance on this point and now advises that "it's usually safe to eat sushi and other dishes made with raw fish when you're pregnant."

Smoked salmon is another matter, however, because it can contain *Listeria*, a bacterium that thrives at refrigeration temperatures and is commonly found in meats and seafood with a long refrigerated shelf life. Because *Listeria* can be quite dangerous during pregnancy, you should avoid smoked salmon unless it is heated before serving. *Listeria* is relatively easy to kill with heat, so it's safe to add smoked salmon and deli meats to anything cooked, such as quiche or frittatas.

Omega-3s and Postpartum Depression

The postpartum phase may seem a long way off, and the likelihood of being impacted by depression during that time is quite low. Even so, it's worth learning a little about the topic now, because you may be able to further lower the odds of developing postpartum depression by optimizing your intake of specific omega-3 fats during pregnancy.

Given the importance of omega-3 fats to brain health, it has long been suspected that a deficiency could play a role in postpartum depression. We know that a mother's own supply of omega-3 fats often becomes depleted during pregnancy, as the baby soaks up these important fatty acids at a rapid pace. Researchers have suggested that this depletion could compromise the mother's production of feel-good brain chemicals.

Somewhat surprisingly, the types of omega-3 fatty acids found in fish oil don't seem to have much impact. In most studies on this subject, fish oil intake during pregnancy does not significantly reduce the likelihood of developing postpartum depression or reduce the severity of symptoms.[20]

Yet new research points to a different form of omega-3, called alpha-linolenic acid (ALA). Found in nuts, seeds, and plant-based oils, this form appears to be much more useful for preventing postpartum depression. One study found that when women took a supplement with ALA starting in midpregnancy, only 12% had a score indicative of significant postpartum depression in the months after delivery, compared to 22% for women taking either fish oil or no omega-3 supplement.[21] Fortunately, it's generally not necessary to add a separate supplement to get enough ALA. It can be found in large amounts in several foods—namely flax seeds and flax seed oil, chia seeds, hemp seeds, walnuts, and canola oil.

In the study, the amount of ALA taken was 2.4 grams per day, which can be found in one tablespoon of ground flax seeds, one teaspoon of flax seed oil, 14 walnut halves, or three tablespoons of hemp seeds. You don't need to consume these foods every day to make a difference. The goal is merely to include more foods rich in ALA over the course of the week. That could mean having chia seed pudding for breakfast or dessert some days, adding a tablespoon of flax oil to salad dressings, and snacking on flax seed crackers or walnuts. These small additions to your diet now could have significant benefits down the line, allowing you to have an easier time after you deliver.

Key Points

- Higher intake of omega-3 fats during pregnancy appears to reduce the odds of preterm birth, support infant brain development, and potentially reduce the odds of your child developing asthma or food allergies.

- To reap the full benefits of omega-3 fats, choose a good-quality fish oil supplement providing at least 500 milligrams of DHA, plus at least some EPA.

- If you're vegetarian or vegan, look for an omega-3 supplement made from algae oil, such as Nordic Naturals Algae Omega.

- Alternatively, you can get enough omega-3 fats by eating lower-mercury cold-water fish, such as salmon, at least two to three times per week.

- Good-quality sushi made from low-mercury fish is fairly safe, but given concerns over *Listeria*, smoked salmon should be avoided unless cooked.

- To reduce the odds of developing postpartum depression, include more foods high in the omega-3 fat ALA, which is found in flax seeds, flax seed oil, hemp and chia seeds, and walnuts.

Chapter 3

Vitamin D, Calcium, and Magnesium

THE LATEST RESEARCH on vitamin D has revealed two surprising trends. The first is the profound impact that vitamin D can have on reducing the chance of preterm birth and other pregnancy complications. The second is the wide gulf between the vitamin D level usually considered adequate and the level that is optimal during pregnancy.

Researchers were originally suspicious that vitamin D could play an important role in pregnancy because of the clear racial disparity in rates of premature birth. Regardless of income levels, Black infants are twice as likely to be born premature.[1] It's also well known that race impacts vitamin D levels. People with darker skin tones need significantly more UV exposure to produce the same amount of vitamin D, which increases the odds of a deficiency. One study of pregnant women in Pittsburgh found that Black women were six times more likely to have a severe vitamin D deficiency than white women.[2]

Noticing this pattern, researchers began to investigate whether there may be a link between vitamin D levels and premature birth. It quickly became apparent that the two are connected, with one early observational study reporting a 47% lower rate of preterm birth in women who had optimal vitamin D levels in the third trimester.[3]

Inspired by these early findings, doctors and researchers at a hospital in South Carolina initiated a new, experimental standard of care for pregnant women that included routine vitamin D testing and free high-dose supplements. Doctors gave patients personalized dosing recommendations based on their current vitamin D levels, with the goal of raising levels to more than 40 nanograms per milliliter (ng/mL) or 100 nanomoles per Liter (nmol/L).[4] This is significantly higher than the level normally considered sufficient, which is 20 ng/mL.

The results of the experiment were dramatic, showing that the women who were able to get their vitamin D level above 40 ng/mL had a 60% lower risk of preterm birth.[5] One explanation for this extraordinary effect is that vitamin D regulates the immune system, both reducing inflammation and boosting immunity to infection.[6] In follow-up studies, numerous groups of researchers have shown a clear link between higher vitamin D levels and lower odds of premature birth.[7] Even so, not every study has demonstrated the same benefits seen in the South Carolina study, likely because the doses were far too low.[8]

A typical vitamin D supplement provides 600–1,000 IU, but to reach the level associated with the lowest odds of preterm birth and other pregnancy complications, most women need at least 4,000 IU per day. In a randomized trial published in the prestigious *Journal of the American Medical Association* (*JAMA*), a dose of 4,000 IU per day during pregnancy was found to raise the average vitamin D level close to our benchmark of 40 ng/mL, but a quarter of the women were still deficient, with levels below 30 ng/mL.[9] This variation may be due to differences in how various forms of vitamin D supplements are absorbed, as well as genetic differences between individuals.[10]

Given that people respond differently to vitamin D supplements, one option is to start with a conservative dose of approximately 4,000 IU per day, in addition to the amount in your prenatal, then test your vitamin D level after one or two months. You can then adjust the dose if needed. For those with a significant deficiency, the Endocrine Society guidelines recommend treatment with 6,000 IU of vitamin D per day for two weeks, followed by a lower ongoing maintenance dose.[11]

These amounts are in line with the recommendation of Dr. Cedric Garland, one of the world's leading authorities on vitamin D. He suggests that people with a deficiency usually need to take 5,000–10,000 IU per day, which is equivalent to what we would naturally produce from ten to twenty minutes of midday sun exposure in summer.[12]

You can also try to raise your vitamin D levels by spending time in the sun each day, but only if you live in the right part of the world. In cold climates, the sun is rarely strong enough in winter to generate sufficient vitamin D. As Dr. Garland notes, "In Boston, you cannot make any vitamin D from

November through March, even if you were standing naked in the middle of the city."

When choosing a supplement, the preferred form is vitamin D3, which is more effective than vitamin D2.[13] It's also best to choose an oil-based gel capsule or liquid drops and to take the supplement with a meal containing some fat in order to boost absorption.

Maintaining an optimal vitamin D level throughout pregnancy has an array of other benefits, including improved blood sugar control and insulin sensitivity and a lower risk of developing preeclampsia.[14] Having a higher vitamin D level appears to reduce the odds of developing gestational diabetes by almost 30%.[15]

Getting enough vitamin D during pregnancy also helps establish your baby's own stores, with benefits for their bone development and immune system. Numerous studies have found that babies born with higher vitamin D levels are much less likely to develop respiratory infections such as RSV (respiratory syncytial virus).[16]

Maintaining an optimal vitamin D level during pregnancy will give your baby a head start, but they will also need their own vitamin D supplement after they're born. This vitamin plays many critical roles during infancy and early childhood, including building strong bones and calibrating the immune system to protect against allergies and infections. The American Academy of Pediatrics and other advisory groups recommend giving babies 400 IU per day, starting in the first few days after birth. This is discussed in further detail in Chapter 20.

Calcium and Magnesium

The final nutrient often lacking in prenatals is calcium. Calcium requirements increase dramatically during the second and third trimesters, when vast amounts are needed to support your baby's rapid bone growth. Nature has decided that if calcium is in short supply during this time, the baby comes first: calcium will be pulled from the mother's teeth and bones, potentially causing dental problems and a loss of bone mineral density that can last long after delivery, increasing the risk of fractures.

To combat this issue, the American College of Obstetricians and Gynecologists (ACOG) recommends a minimum intake of 1,300 milligrams of calcium per day during pregnancy. To put this into context, one cup of milk or yogurt contains approximately 300 milligrams, so you would need several servings of dairy per day to reach the recommended intake. The richest nondairy sources of calcium are tofu, navy beans, and leafy greens, but these foods also contain compounds known as oxalates, which reduce calcium absorption.

If you eat multiple servings of dairy each day and take a prenatal that contains some calcium, you may be getting close to the recommended amount, but it's easy to fall short. On average, pregnant women get a little over half the amount needed, or around 700–800 milligrams of calcium per day.[17]

Given this, it usually makes sense to add a separate calcium supplement to your regime, at least during the second and third trimesters. The recommended dose is 400–600 milligrams per day if you eat dairy, or 1,000 milligrams if you don't.

Ensuring that you get enough calcium during the second half of pregnancy has a range of benefits beyond simply protecting your bone health and supporting your baby's growth. For reasons that are not well understood, calcium is associated with a significantly lower risk of preterm birth.[18] It also helps prevent high blood pressure, likely by improving the ability of blood vessels to expand and contract when needed and by preventing excess fluid retention. By helping to regulate blood pressure in this way, calcium is one of the most effective ways to lower the odds of developing preeclampsia. Randomized studies have seen a 50% drop in cases among women taking extra calcium during the second half of pregnancy.[19]

The potential to have such a profound impact on maternal health with a relatively simple measure led the Bill and Melinda Gates Foundation to fund large-scale studies on the topic, including a recent study of more than 20,000 pregnant women in India and Africa. The findings, published in the *New England Journal of Medicine* in 2024, confirmed that taking 500 milligrams of calcium per day is just as effective as higher doses when it comes to preventing preeclampsia.[20] In women starting with a very low-calcium diet, a higher-dose supplement is even more effective at reducing the odds of preterm birth.

Getting enough calcium during pregnancy undoubtedly has a range of benefits, but side effects can sometimes become an obstacle. Most standard calcium supplements are in the form of calcium carbonate, which can slow digestion and cause constipation, particularly during pregnancy. To avoid these side effects, look for a supplement that contains calcium malate or calcium citrate.

Another option is to choose a supplement that combines calcium and magnesium. Although studies have found little evidence of a need to supplement with magnesium during pregnancy, many women are mildly deficient, and addressing this can reduce headaches, insomnia, constipation, muscle spasms, and anxiety.

One of the most effective forms for all these purposes is magnesium citrate, whereas magnesium glycinate is most helpful for sleep. For treating muscle pain, magnesium malate is the preferred form. If you are prone to headaches or migraines, taking magnesium and additional riboflavin every day may help. A 2023 study found that this combination reduced the frequency and severity of migraines in 77% of pregnant women.[21] The best form of magnesium for this purpose is magnesium L-threonate.

Because calcium can reduce the absorption of iron, it's better to take your prenatal in the morning and your calcium and magnesium supplements at night. Vitamin D can be taken at any time but is best absorbed with a meal. One of the many benefits of vitamin D is that it improves our ability to absorb calcium from food and supplements, but vitamin D does not need to be taken at the same time as calcium to have this effect.

Key Points

- Ensuring adequate vitamin D levels during pregnancy can significantly reduce the risk of preterm birth, likely by reducing inflammation and preventing infections.

- The optimal vitamin D level for preventing preterm birth is at least 40 ng/mL.

- To reach this level, most people need to supplement with at least 4,000 IU per day. Follow-up testing can help determine whether you need an even higher dose.

- Babies should typically be given 400 IU per day of vitamin D starting soon after birth.

- Calcium is vital for protecting your bone health and reducing the odds of preterm birth and preeclampsia.

- During the second and third trimesters, most people need to take an additional 400–600 milligrams of calcium per day. Calcium citrate and calcium malate are the preferred forms.

- Taking a combination of calcium and magnesium may help with common pregnancy ailments, including muscle pain, insomnia, and headaches.

Chapter 4

Aspirin, Preeclampsia, and Placenta Health

O NE AREA IN which conventional medical advice often falls short is the prevention of preeclampsia. Some doctors proactively inform their patients about ways to avoid this condition, but many do not. Countless women are never told that a few simple measures may improve the odds of a healthier and easier pregnancy.

Preeclampsia is a common condition characterized by high blood pressure that appears after 20 weeks of pregnancy. Although high blood pressure is the main symptom, preeclampsia often causes dysfunction of the kidneys and other organs. One of the first signs is usually elevated liver enzymes. Preeclampsia impacts 1 in 30 pregnancies, but it's much more common in those who are pregnant after IVF, are over the age of 35, or who have a high BMI or gestational diabetes.[1]

Even though the condition is quite common, treatment options have not progressed much over the past century. If high blood pressure reaches a concerning level and medication is not effective, the solution is typically an early induction or C-section.

Fortunately, science has come a long way in identifying the potential risk factors and revealing effective ways to reduce the odds of developing preeclampsia in the first place. This provides an opportunity to get ahead of the issue and give babies a greater chance of making it to a full-term delivery.

Preventing preeclampsia can also have long-term benefits for your own health. Although the world of maternal medicine is often laser focused on the end goal of having a healthy baby, a mother's health after delivery matters, too, although it rarely receives the attention it deserves. This is troubling because preeclampsia can leave a lasting impact on a mother's heart and circulatory system, setting the stage for issues such as high blood pressure that may continue long after delivery.[2]

The most recent studies have revealed that having high blood pressure for a sustained length of time during pregnancy can cause subtle changes to the mother's heart. The chronically increased workload leads to a thickening of the heart walls, which can compromise the ability to pump blood effectively and lead to ongoing high blood pressure.[3] The net result is often postpartum hypertension, a condition that impacts more than a quarter of women who experience high blood pressure or preeclampsia during pregnancy.[4]

The best solution is to determine whether you have any risk factors for preeclampsia and, if so, to take action earlier in pregnancy to reduce the chance of this problem occurring. This is worthwhile not only for protecting your baby's health and preventing premature delivery but also for safeguarding your own long-term health and ensuring an easier postpartum recovery.

Why Age and IVF Matter

Age 35 is considered a watershed milestone in the world of obstetrics. Pregnancies after that point are officially labeled as "advanced maternal age" (AMA) and subject to different treatment recommendations. In reality, the risks are not that much greater when you cross the threshold from 34 to 35, but there is a slow and gradual rise in the chance of complications starting in the early 30s and increasing more sharply after age 40. The odds of developing preeclampsia, for example, double after age 40.[5]

There is also a higher risk of preeclampsia in IVF pregnancies, particularly after frozen embryo transfers, and in women with PCOS, diabetes, or autoimmune conditions such as lupus.[6] The common thread in all these risk factors is the function of the placenta.

The placenta is a critical interface between the mother's and baby's blood supply. The maternal side of this interface is made up of the cells of the uterine lining and specialized blood vessels known as spiral arteries. Before pregnancy, the spiral arteries provide oxygen and nutrients to the uterine lining. During pregnancy, they undergo a major structural change to provide blood flow to the placenta.

This change begins in the earliest stage of pregnancy. Cells from the outer layer of the embryo burrow into the uterine lining and send signals to the mother's blood vessels to change shape and widen, thus providing increased blood flow.

If you are over 35, this process can be impaired. Your spiral arteries may be more stubborn—they may not change and widen as much as normal, which reduces blood flow to the placenta.[7] Although this doesn't normally cause problems, in rare cases it can compromise the placenta's ability to meet the baby's needs toward the end of the third trimester, when the demand for oxygen and nutrients reaches its peak. When poor blood flow is detected, the placenta sends out chemical signals to tell the mother's circulatory system to increase blood pressure, potentially leading to preeclampsia.

A similar issue can sometimes occur in IVF pregnancies, particularly those conceived after a frozen embryo transfer. One plausible explanation is that the medication protocols used for embryo transfer don't fully replicate all the important hormones and growth factors produced during natural ovulation that trigger changes to blood vessels and prepare the uterine lining for implantation. If the uterine lining is less receptive and the mother's blood vessels don't receive the same signals to prepare for pregnancy, this may compromise the formation of a good connection between the mother's and baby's blood supply. The mother's blood vessels may not undergo the same changes to create strong blood flow to the placenta, which may in turn increase the likelihood of preeclampsia.[8]

This is not a major cause for concern because the chance of developing preeclampsia in an IVF pregnancy or after the age of 35 is still less than 10%. However, it does mean that your placenta may need a little help to function optimally, and you may need closer monitoring toward the end of your pregnancy.[9]

The same may be true if you have another health issue that can increase blood clotting or impair blood flow through the placenta. These issues include a high BMI, PCOS, diabetes, lupus, or a history of multiple miscarriages due to immune factors.[10]

Even if you have several of these risk factors, the odds of any complication occurring is still relatively low, and your baby is likely to be perfectly healthy. Nevertheless, taking proactive steps may lower the risks even further by supporting the health of your placenta and reducing inflammation.

We've already covered some of the most effective strategies for doing so, namely making sure you get enough vitamin D, omega-3 fatty acids, and calcium. In women with a particularly high risk of developing preeclampsia, supplementing with magnesium may also improve the odds.[11] Another strategy with clear support in the scientific research, and a focus of this chapter, is taking low-dose aspirin.

The Benefits of Aspirin

The rationale behind using aspirin to prevent preeclampsia and improve the health of the placenta is based on its ability to reduce inflammation in blood vessels and prevent the formation of unwanted blood clots. These effects seem to translate into improved blood flow through the placenta, which reduces the odds of developing preeclampsia and other complications.[12]

In years past, the American College of Obstetricians and Gynecologists (ACOG) recommended aspirin only to women who had experienced preeclampsia in a prior pregnancy, as this is associated with a 40% chance of recurrence. Today's guidelines recommend aspirin more widely and encompass individuals with at least one of the high-risk factors or more than one of the moderate-risk factors.

The high-risk factors include:

- a history of preeclampsia
- being pregnant with multiples
- kidney disease
- autoimmune disease
- type 1 or type 2 diabetes
- chronic hypertension

The moderate-risk factors include:

- being pregnant for the first time
- being over 35 years old
- having a BMI over 30
- having a family history of preeclampsia
- being African American
- having a prior pregnancy complication

In the United States, more than 85% of pregnancies have either one of the high-risk factors or multiple moderate-risk factors.[13] The most recent data indicates that having PCOS or conceiving by IVF should also be added to the list, taking the percentage of pregnancies where aspirin should be recommended to well over 90%.[14]

If you fall into this very large category, taking aspirin at a specific stage of pregnancy may cancel out much of the increased risk. Numerous randomized studies have shown that aspirin dramatically lowers the chance of developing pre-eclampsia.[15] By supporting the health of the placenta, aspirin may also help prevent preterm birth and fetal-growth restriction.[16] But timing is important. Studies have indicated that aspirin is effective only if started before 16 weeks, ideally at around 11 or 12 weeks.

Starting aspirin after 16 weeks doesn't seem to convey much benefit. This may be because most of the changes to the blood vessels have already occurred by that time.

That doesn't mean that sooner is always better, however. In the early 2000s, IVF clinics started recommending aspirin following embryo transfer, with the hope of increasing the chance of implantation and reducing the odds of miscarriage. It's still in doubt whether aspirin can make much difference in achieving those goals,[17] but after this practice started, two perceptive obstetricians noticed a new trend: fertility patients taking aspirin right from the start of pregnancy were much more likely to have a certain type of bleeding during pregnancy, called a subchorionic hematoma (SCH).[18]

This bleeding, which is thought to occur due to small tears in blood vessels between the placenta and uterine wall, appears to be much more common in women taking aspirin in early pregnancy. [19] One study reported that 40–50% of women who conceived through IVF and took aspirin throughout the first trimester developed an SCH, compared to 10% of those not taking aspirin.[20]

The chance that an SCH will lead to a more serious complication is low.[21] If the size of the SCH compared to that of the placenta is very large, and if it forms before 7 weeks, there may be a higher chance of miscarriage, but this is the exception, not the rule.[22] Most often, an SCH resolves on its own without issue.[23] Even so, the unexpected and heavy bleeding that can occur with an SCH often causes a great deal of stress.

To avoid this situation, it is likely better to delay starting aspirin until around 12 weeks, unless your doctor advises otherwise. Your doctor may recommend aspirin throughout the first trimester if you have a history of miscarriage due to immune issues or blood clotting. In these situations, the benefits of taking aspirin in the first trimester may outweigh the risk of developing an SCH, although the evidence is unclear.[24] It's also worth noting that heparin, another blood-thinning medication used to minimize blood clotting in those with a history of recurrent miscarriage, appears to be much more effective for that purpose and doesn't seem to impact the chance of developing an SCH.[25]

If you decide to take aspirin, the usual dose is 80–160 milligrams per day in the form of a low-dose or baby aspirin tablet. In the United States, where a low-dose aspirin tablet is typically 81 milligrams, some doctors recommend two tablets per day for higher-risk patients. One tablet per day may be sufficient if you have only minor risk factors for preeclampsia.

Aspirin is usually stopped at some point before 36 weeks out of a concern that it may contribute to bleeding risks around the time of delivery. The impact on bleeding is relatively small, but there is also little benefit to continuing aspirin during the third trimester. We know this from a randomized clinical trial, published in 2023 in *JAMA*, which found that in women at high risk of developing preeclampsia, continuing aspirin until delivery or stopping at 24–28 weeks made virtually no difference.[26] The most useful time frame for taking aspirin therefore seems to be weeks 12–24.

Although aspirin is considered very safe, individuals with a sensitivity to salicylates may react negatively. Symptoms may include ringing in the ears, asthma, bladder irritation, muscle pain, and nasal polyps. You may notice these symptoms when consuming foods that are high in natural salicylates, such as mint, spices, tea, and berries. If you have salicylate sensitivity, it may be better to skip aspirin and instead rely on the strategies discussed in earlier chapters, namely increasing your intake of vitamin D, omega-3 fats, calcium, and possibly magnesium. In addition, aspirin is typically not recommended if you have a history of stomach ulcers or stomach bleeding.

Other Strategies for Supporting Placenta Health

Although taking aspirin and the supplements discussed in earlier chapters can significantly reduce your odds of developing preeclampsia, it is not possible to prevent every case. If you end up developing high blood pressure or preeclampsia despite your best efforts, or if you are at a higher risk because of preeclampsia in a prior pregnancy, a supplement that may prove helpful is L-arginine.

This amino acid increases the natural production of nitric oxide, which signals blood vessels to widen, thereby increasing blood flow. Studies have found that in women with preeclampsia, supplementing with L-arginine lowers blood pressure and reduces the need for medication.[27] It is also helpful for prevention. One study of high-risk pregnancies found that supplementing with L-arginine starting at 20 weeks was associated with a much lower chance of developing preeclampsia. In the control group, 23% developed preeclampsia, compared to just 6% of those taking L-arginine.[28] By improving blood flow through the placenta, L-arginine can also minimize fetal growth restriction.[29] A typical dose is 3 grams per day and it is most effective when taken in weeks 20–28.[30]

Exercise is also helpful for preventing and managing preeclampsia. Although the data is somewhat inconsistent, several studies have reported that regular walking can reduce the odds of developing the condition by 20–30%.[31] Stretching may be even more effective, with one study finding that just 3% of women following a stretching program developed preeclampsia, compared to 15% of those who walked regularly.[32] One explanation for this effect is that stretching promotes the release of natural chemicals that reduce inflammation, lower the heart rate, and help blood vessels relax.

Yoga is likely to have the same benefits. Practicing yoga just once a week has been found to significantly reduce blood pressure in women with mild preeclampsia.[33] A randomized study of women with major risk factors for the condition also found that practicing yoga in the second and third trimesters significantly reduced the chance of developing high blood pressure.[34]

Key Points

- If you are over 35, conceived through IVF, or have a higher BMI or certain other risk factors, taking low-dose aspirin may support the health of your placenta and reduce the odds of developing preeclampsia.

- The optimal time frame for taking aspirin is in weeks 12–24.

- The recommended dose is 80–160 milligrams per day.

- If you end up developing high blood pressure or pre-eclampsia, or if you had preeclampsia in a prior pregnancy, it may also be worth supplementing with L-arginine at a dose of 3 grams per day.

- Exercise, particularly stretching and yoga, may also help lower blood pressure and prevent preeclampsia.

Chapter 5

Myo-Inositol for Gestational Diabetes

L IKE SO MANY other areas of pregnancy health, the conventional approach to gestational diabetes involves waiting until the condition is diagnosed and then trying to address the consequences through either medications or an early C-section. A more proactive approach is to consider whether you may have higher odds of developing this condition and, if so, focusing on prevention and improving insulin sensitivity.

Gestational diabetes is a common condition that impacts at least one in 20 pregnancies. It is even more common in women who are over 35 or have PCOS, a high BMI, or a family history of diabetes. Fortunately, the scientific research provides clear guidance on strategies to prevent and manage this condition.

One of the most effective approaches is taking the supplement myo-inositol. This sugar molecule can significantly improve insulin function and blood sugar levels, which in turn helps protect both your baby's health and your own health.

What Causes Gestational Diabetes?

Although the precise cause of gestational diabetes is not entirely clear, the most likely explanation is that it occurs because pregnancy hormones make insulin less effective. Insulin's primary job is to tell cells in the liver and muscles to soak up glucose from the bloodstream. During the second and third trimesters, hormones from the placenta make the mother's cells less sensitive to this message from insulin, creating a mild form of insulin resistance.[1] Most women can simply make more insulin to get around this problem, but if you already have another factor contributing to insulin resistance, such as PCOS, genetics, or a higher BMI, it's more difficult to counteract the blocking effect of pregnancy hormones on insulin function.

If your cells can't properly respond to insulin, blood glucose remains high, which can lead to a range of downstream consequences during pregnancy. One of the main concerns is a higher chance of needing a C-section due to the baby's size. Gestational diabetes is also associated with a higher chance of preterm birth and preeclampsia.[2]

Assessing the Odds

The risk factors for developing gestational diabetes fall into two broad categories. The first includes anyone with PCOS, a BMI over 30, a history of gestational diabetes in a previous pregnancy, or a family history of diabetes. For these individuals, the odds of developing the condition are at least three times higher than average. If you fall into this category, it's likely worth taking active steps to improve insulin sensitivity before a problem arises by starting myo-inositol in the first or second trimester.

The second category is more of a gray area. For individuals who are over age 35, are pregnant with multiples, or have a BMI over 25, the odds of developing gestational diabetes are roughly two times higher than average. If you fall into this category, it's reasonable to wait until the results of your glucose tolerance test are available to see how your insulin function performs. This test is normally performed between 24 and 28 weeks. If the results indicate that you're having difficulty managing your blood sugar levels, it will be helpful to start taking myo-inositol at that point. Alternatively, you may decide not to wait for your glucose tolerance test and to start taking myo-inositol at around 20 weeks if you'd prefer to err on the side of prevention.

Age has a surprising impact on the chance of developing gestational diabetes. For reasons not fully understood, the odds steadily increase with each passing year after the age of 18.[3] This increase is even more pronounced in those of Asian descent, so if both age and ethnicity are potential contributing factors for you, there is even greater reason to take active steps to manage blood sugar levels.[4]

You might also consider taking a more proactive approach if you experience signs of insulin resistance, such as unusual hunger, thirst, or fatigue, especially after eating high-carbohydrate foods.

How Myo-Inositol Helps

Myo-inositol is a naturally occurring sugar molecule found in small amounts in foods such as nuts, fruit, and beans. The body uses myo-inositol to produce other compounds called inositol phosphoglycans (IPGs), which activate the transporters that let glucose into cells. In this respect, IPGs act in a similar way to how insulin lowers blood sugar levels by moving it out of the bloodstream and into cells, where it can be stored or used for energy. Myo-inositol can therefore counteract insulin resistance and prevent spikes in blood glucose.

Myo-inositol has been used for many years to improve fertility in those with PCOS, a condition characterized by insulin resistance. By improving insulin and glucose levels, it helps rebalance the hormonal issues associated with PCOS, which often restores ovulation and makes it easier to get pregnant.[5] The natural extension of this—using myo-inositol to continue managing insulin function in pregnancy—began with a chance discovery by doctors in Italy. They noticed that when women with PCOS continued taking myo-inositol during pregnancy, they were much less likely to develop gestational diabetes.[6]

This led researchers to ask whether the supplement could also help prevent gestational diabetes in other high-risk groups. The answer was a clear yes. Placebo-controlled trials demonstrated that myo-inositol more than halves the risk of developing gestational diabetes.[7]

Myo-inositol also reduces the severity of the condition by improving insulin sensitivity and lowering blood glucose levels.[8] This has many subsequent benefits, including a lower rate of preeclampsia and preterm birth, less need for insulin, fewer babies who are large for their gestational age, and fewer episodes of low blood sugar in newborns.[9]

The typical dose of myo-inositol is two grams, twice per day, for a total of four grams per day. (Studies using a lower dose of just one gram per day found little benefit.[10]) It can be started at any point during pregnancy after checking with your doctor. Considering the dosage, many people find the powdered form more convenient than taking several capsules. You can take the supplement with or without food. It often improves sleep when taken at bedtime.[11]

Although myo-inositol appears to be one of the most effective ways to prevent and manage gestational diabetes, other supplements can also make a difference.

Vitamin D is useful because it helps the body both produce and use insulin, thereby improving the ability of cells to absorb glucose.[12] As a result, women with higher levels of vitamin D at the beginning of pregnancy are much less likely to develop gestational diabetes.[13]

Supplementing with vitamin D can also improve blood sugar control in those who already have gestational diabetes.[14] One study found that supplementing with the equivalent of 3,500 IU per day could significantly improve insulin resistance in pregnant women.[15]

Fish oil has also shown benefits, likely because omega-3 fats can boost the production of insulin and improve insulin sensitivity.[16] In one double-blind study of women with gestational diabetes, supplementing with fish oil significantly reduced the rate of newborn complications. The percentage of babies with jaundice, for example, dropped from 33% to 8%.[17]

Combining vitamin D and fish oil appears to produce even better results, with a significant reduction in fasting glucose levels and insulin resistance.[18]

Beyond supplements, it's also possible to improve blood sugar control through simple lifestyle changes. Studies have shown that minimizing sugar and processed carbohydrates and switching to carbohydrates that are higher in fiber and broken down more slowly can improve blood sugar control.[19] The best choices are legumes, nuts, seeds, unprocessed grains, and vegetables. You can also prevent spikes in blood sugar by pairing carbohydrates with fat and protein to slow the release of glucose.

Staying physically active is another good way to improve blood-sugar control. Walking or exercising after meals is particularly helpful for reducing potential glucose spikes. In addition, resistance training can build up muscle mass, which improves the ability of muscles to respond to insulin and absorb glucose from the bloodstream.[20]

Using some combination of these strategies to manage your blood sugar can not only significantly reduce the rate of pregnancy complications but will also help you feel better, with steady energy levels, better sleep, and even a possible improvement in pregnancy nausea.[21] (For more on how managing blood sugar can lessen nausea, see Chapter 11).

Key Points

- If you have PCOS, a BMI over 30, or a family history of diabetes, or if you experienced gestational diabetes in a previous pregnancy, taking myo-inositol can likely halve your risk of developing gestational diabetes.

- Myo-inositol is also worth considering if you are over 35, are pregnant with multiples, or have a BMI over 25, although if you fall into this category, it's reasonable to wait until your glucose tolerance test to find out how your insulin function responds to pregnancy.

- If you do develop gestational diabetes, continuing with myo-inositol can help protect your baby from high glucose levels and reduce the odds of other complications.

- The typical dose is two grams, twice per day.

- Choosing unprocessed and high-fiber carbohydrates can improve blood sugar control, as can regular walking and resistance training.

Chapter 6

Miscarriage Supplements and Progesterone

I F YOU'VE BEEN following the miscarriage supplement plan in my earlier book *It Starts with the Egg*, you can likely trim your supplement regime now that you're pregnant. The supplements covered in that book are most helpful before you conceive because they generally aim to prevent chromosomal abnormalities in the developing egg. These abnormalities, which occur spontaneously as an egg or sperm matures, are the single most common cause of miscarriage, accounting for at least 50% of early pregnancy losses.[1] By supporting cellular energy production in the months before ovulation, supplements such as coenzyme Q10 (CoQ10) and N-acetylcysteine (NAC) can improve the odds of an egg having enough cellular energy to process chromosomes correctly. Once you're pregnant, this work is done, meaning most of the supplements are no longer needed.

The situation is slightly different if you've experienced a miscarriage due to immune or clotting issues rather than genetic abnormalities in the embryo. In that situation, there may be value in continuing with certain supplements in order to reduce blood clotting and modulate the immune system.

Although chromosomal errors are the most common cause of miscarriage, the younger you are and the more miscarriages you've had, the more likely the cause relates to issues with the immune system, an infection, hormones, or blood clotting rather than a genetic error in the embryo. Testing for some of these issues is covered in more detail in Chapter 15 of *It Starts with the Egg*. If you suspect an immune or clotting issue, the supplements most likely to help during early pregnancy are CoQ10 and NAC, as the next section explains. If you're not sure what caused your prior pregnancy losses, it's reasonable to take these supplements as a precaution, in case they help.

Another option for those with unexplained recurrent miscarriage is supplementing with progesterone, but as you'll learn later in this chapter, the evidence on that front remains unclear.

CoQ10 and NAC for Miscarriage Prevention

Although the research is quite sparse, preliminary studies indicate that taking CoQ10 during pregnancy may reduce the chance of miscarriage caused by immune issues, particularly antiphospholipid antibody syndrome. When these autoimmune antibodies are present, unwanted immune activity causes oxidative stress and increased blood clotting, which reduces blood flow to the placenta and increases the chance of pregnancy loss.

CoQ10 appears to interrupt this chain of events, reducing blood clotting caused by antiphospholipid antibodies.[2] In one study demonstrating these beneficial effects, the dose used was 200 milligrams per day of ubiquinol (the reduced form of CoQ10). A similar dose of standard CoQ10 likely has similar effects.

Another study reported that CoQ10 can improve some of the other immune imbalances often seen in those with recurrent pregnancy loss. It does this by restoring the balance between two groups of T-cells, known as Th1 and Th2 cells. In effect, CoQ10 shifts the immune system toward a less inflammatory state.[3]

Although the use of CoQ10 during pregnancy has not been studied extensively, it is naturally produced by our cells in increasing amounts throughout pregnancy, indicating that it's likely safe to take during this time. Levels typically rise with each trimester, and when this rise does not occur, there seems to be an increased chance of pregnancy loss.[4]

If you have a history of miscarriage due to immune or clotting issues, it's likely worth continuing 200 milligrams of CoQ10 through at least the first trimester (after checking with your doctor). It's also reasonable to take this supplement even if you're not sure of the cause of your pregnancy losses. It may help, and there appears to be little downside.

Preliminary research also suggests potential value in taking NAC, an amino-acid derivative that helps support our natural antioxidant defenses. In one small study of women with unexplained recurrent miscarriage, NAC significantly increased the chance of carrying to term. Pregnancy continued past 15 weeks in 73% of the women taking NAC, compared to 20% in the group not taking it.[5] This isolated finding should be treated with some skepticism until it is repeated by other researchers. Even so, several studies outside the pregnancy context have found that NAC reduces both inflammation and the activity of blood-clotting factors, which provides a plausible explanation for the reduction in miscarriage risk.[6]

Another theory is that some cases of miscarriage may involve oxidative damage to the placenta.[7] NAC may help address this problem by increasing production of glutathione, the master antioxidant that normally serves to protect the placenta from oxidation.

Although NAC has not been studied extensively in pregnancy, it is generally considered safe. It's the treatment of choice for acetaminophen/paracetamol overdose in pregnancy and is routinely used for this purpose.[8]

Several randomized studies have also reported that NAC is safe and effective for treating pregnancy complications involving inflammation of the amniotic sac due to infection.[9] One study gave NAC to women who were treated for bacterial vaginosis during pregnancy and found a significant reduction in the chance of preterm birth. On average, the women taking NAC carried to 37.4 weeks, compared to 34.1 weeks in the group treated with antibiotics alone.[10]

Nevertheless, little research has been done on the daily use of NAC in early pregnancy, so it's a personal decision whether to take this supplement. NAC is most likely to be worthwhile if you've had multiple miscarriages without any known cause. The typical dose is 600 mg per day. It can be taken at any time, although it's gentler on the stomach if taken with food.

Progesterone for Recurrent Miscarriage

Progesterone is a hormone that plays an integral role in early pregnancy. It thickens and modifies the uterine lining to allow an embryo to successfully implant, helps reorganize blood vessels to provide nutrients to a growing embryo, and calms the immune system, preventing unwanted immune reactions. Given these important roles, one might expect that anyone who has experienced a pregnancy loss should have progesterone levels monitored in early pregnancy to ensure that this hormone is maintained at optimal levels. Unfortunately, the research in this area is contradictory, and there are no clear answers as to when progesterone testing and treatment will be worthwhile. Overall, checking your progesterone is most likely to be helpful if you're still very early in your pregnancy and have previously had several unexplained losses.

In a naturally conceived pregnancy, progesterone is made in the ovaries by the collection of cells that previously surrounded an egg. After ovulation, these cells form a temporary structure called the corpus luteum, which starts making a small amount of progesterone to prepare the uterine lining for pregnancy. If pregnancy occurs, the hormone hCG (human chorionic gonadotropin), which is produced by the newly forming placenta, sends a message to the corpus luteum to increase progesterone production, which it continues to do until the placenta takes over the job. The placenta begins making progesterone at around 4 to 5 weeks and completely takes over by around 8 to 10 weeks.

In an IVF pregnancy, there is typically no corpus luteum to make progesterone because an embryo is usually transferred after an egg retrieval cycle or artificial cycle rather than during natural ovulation. To make up for this deficit, progesterone is given in the form of injections or vaginal gel, usually starting shortly before transfer and continuing until long past the point when the placenta normally takes over.

This long progesterone treatment in IVF patients is probably unnecessary, but most clinics would rather err on the side of caution than risk a pregnancy loss from low progesterone, even though little evidence exists that such extended treatment makes any difference.[11] In naturally conceived pregnancies, the situation is quite different, and doctors are much less proactive. Some OBs may order a test during the first trimester and prescribe progesterone to correct low levels, but this is far from the norm. Patient requests for progesterone are often met with strong resistance.

Many OBs are not enthusiastic about progesterone testing and treatment because of the disappointing results of two large, randomized studies. These studies found that giving vaginal progesterone gel to women with a history of recurrent miscarriage has minimal impact on the risk of pregnancy loss.[12] One of these studies reported that progesterone treatment helped only those who had bleeding during pregnancy and a history of at least three losses; even then, the advantage was minor.[13] Despite these discouraging findings, we still can't entirely rule out a broader benefit. It's possible that progesterone could be more effective if started earlier or given as injections or oral tablets, or if treatment is limited to those who are actually found to have low progesterone.

Studies in the IVF context have been more promising and have suggested that correcting low progesterone at the start of pregnancy could make a real difference. As one example, a 2023 study found that giving extra progesterone to patients who were low at the time of the first pregnancy test could significantly reduce miscarriage rates.[14] Researchers tested progesterone levels at 10 days after transfer, and the women who were below 10.6 ng/mL were divided into two groups—one that received additional progesterone and one that did not. The difference in live birth rates was stark. Women who had a low value on day 10 and did not receive additional progesterone had a live birth rate of just 16%, compared to 82% for the group with a good initial progesterone number and 97% in the women who started with a low value but were given additional progesterone.[15] This study indicates that, at least for IVF pregnancies, it's probably useful to test progesterone levels around the time of the first hCG blood test, although this is not yet standard practice.

We don't yet know whether the same effect would be seen in naturally conceived pregnancies, so the value of testing progesterone outside the IVF context is still uncertain. We do, however, have some clues that link pregnancy loss to low progesterone levels at the very start of naturally conceived pregnancies. Specifically, researchers have observed a drop in progesterone levels at around 11 to 15 days after ovulation in pregnancies that ended in early miscarriage.[16] In many of these cases, progesterone likely dropped because the embryo was not viable, so it was not producing enough hCG to stimulate the corpus luteum to make progesterone. In other words, low progesterone is typically a symptom, not a cause, of early pregnancy loss. But researchers were able to pinpoint some rare examples where progesterone dropped before a decline in hCG, which indicates a problem with progesterone production. These cases might have benefited from progesterone treatment if started early enough, although this is still a matter of conjecture.

We don't yet have clear answers on whether progesterone treatment is worthwhile, but it is most likely to be useful if you have a history of recurrent pregnancy loss and are still very early in your pregnancy. After around 7 weeks, the placenta is likely already making all the progesterone needed.

Accurate testing for progesterone is challenging because levels can fluctuate widely from hour to hour. That means we can't place too much reliance on any one lab value. Even so, many fertility doctors consider 10–15 ng/mL the benchmark during early pregnancy and will prescribe progesterone if your level is below that threshold. This approach is not necessarily supported by clear evidence, but progesterone is considered very safe, and the research indicates there is little drawback to erring on the side of treatment.

Key Points

- Most miscarriage supplements can be stopped when you get a positive pregnancy test.

- If you suspect that immune or clotting issues contributed to prior losses, or if your losses were unexplained, it may be worth continuing with CoQ10 and/or NAC, at least through the first trimester.

- The typical dose of CoQ10 is 200 milligrams per day.

- The typical dose of NAC is 600 milligrams per day.

- The evidence for treating low progesterone is mixed, but it's most likely to be helpful if you are still in the earliest stages of pregnancy.

- For recommended supplement brands, see itstartswiththebump.com/supplements

- For a complete summary of supplements, see the appendix.

PART 2

Lab Tests and Screening

Chapter 7

Optimizing Thyroid Function

IT IS COMMON for thyroid hormones to dip during the first or second trimester, even if your levels were previously normal or well controlled with medication. That is because pregnancy places significant demands on the thyroid gland, and it can't always keep up.

Doctors typically test thyroid function at around 8–12 weeks, but checking your thyroid sooner can help ensure that your baby is getting enough active thyroid hormone during the most critical time.

Thyroid Testing

Thyroid function is most often assessed by measuring the level of thyroid stimulating hormone (TSH), with a higher level indicating an underactive thyroid. Produced by the pituitary gland, TSH signals the thyroid to produce active hormones, specifically triiodothyronine (T3) and thyroxine (T4). When the thyroid gland is underactive and doesn't produce enough of these hormones, the pituitary gland responds by releasing more TSH in an attempt to stimulate the thyroid.

Thyroid function can also be assessed more directly by measuring T3 and T4. Of these, free T4 is likely the more useful value, but it's difficult to measure accurately, and values can vary between different labs.

Most guidelines specify that TSH should be below 4 mIU/L during the first trimester. By this definition, about 2–3% of pregnant women are considered hypothyroid.[1] This threshold misses many borderline cases, however, and it seems the optimal TSH level during pregnancy is likely below 2.5 mIU/L. In addition, free T4 should be at least 0.8 ng/dL or 7.5 pg/mL, or above the range for pregnancy given by the testing laboratory. With these benchmarks, 20–30% of pregnant women have suboptimal thyroid function.[2]

This is problematic because thyroid hormones are vital for supporting the baby's brain development and ensuring proper development of the placenta.[3]

Although the impact of thyroid function on the placenta is rarely discussed, it's clear that thyroid hormones are needed to develop a strong connection between the mother's and baby's blood supply. When the thyroid gland is functioning as it should, this increases production of growth factors that promote the development of new blood vessels.[4] Thyroid hormones also promote changes in the maternal arteries to increase nutrient supply to the placenta. Finally, thyroid hormones reduce inflammation in the placenta by increasing immune-calming mediators.[5] This is critical because when inflammation is kept under control during the first trimester, while new blood vessels are forming and burrowing into the uterine lining, the placenta seems to function more efficiently throughout pregnancy, with improved blood flow. As a result, optimal thyroid function during early pregnancy tends to reduce the odds of various complications related to the placenta. These include pregnancy loss, preeclampsia, fetal growth restriction, and preterm birth.[6]

Even so, many doctors offer thyroid testing only after 10 or 12 weeks—and only then for patients they consider "high risk," namely those with a preexisting thyroid condition or obvious symptoms such as fatigue, excess weight gain, and cold sensitivity. The official guidelines recommend against wider screening because of a lack of evidence. In recent years, however, new data has emerged that weighs in favor of early testing and more proactive treatment.[7] Standard practice has just been slow to catch up.

In one of the most compelling recent studies, a group of women had their thyroid function tested at 8 weeks and were treated with levothyroxine (the generic name for Synthroid) if their TSH levels were above 2.5 mIU/L or free T4 below 7.5 pg/mL. Starting this treatment before 9 weeks was found to dramatically reduce a range of complications, including miscarriage, preterm birth, gestational diabetes, preeclampsia, and fetal growth restriction.[8] Most of these complications were reduced by almost 30%, and the rate of pregnancy loss before 12 weeks was reduced by more than 40%. These benefits were minimal or not seen at all when treatment was started between 10 and 24 weeks of pregnancy.

This research tells us that when obstetricians test thyroid hormones for the first time at 10–12 weeks, it is unsurprising that treating borderline cases has minimal effect on the rate of complications. Treatment is starting too late, missing the key time frame when thyroid hormones can support development of a healthy placenta.

A natural increase in T4 occurs at around 7–11 weeks, which researchers think may be a critical window of time when thyroid hormones are most important. By ensuring that thyroid hormone function is optimal during this period, we're setting the stage for a healthier pregnancy.

For this reason, it is useful to have your TSH and T4 tested as soon as you can. If you're still very early in the first trimester or your results are borderline, it may be worth testing again after four to six weeks. If at any point your TSH is above 2.5 mIU/L or your free T4 is below 7.5 pg/mL, it's probably worth asking your doctor about starting Synthroid or increasing your current dose.

Treatment is even more likely to be helpful if you also test positive for thyroid antibodies. In developed countries, where table salt is iodized and women take prenatals containing iodine, the most common cause of low thyroid function is autoimmunity. This occurs when the immune system generates antibodies that interfere with thyroid function.

If your thyroid hormone levels are only slightly abnormal but you also have thyroid antibodies, there is even more reason to start medication. The guidelines advise that treatment "should be considered" in pregnant women with borderline hypothyroidism and positive antibodies, based on a higher risk of preterm delivery and possibly a higher risk of miscarriage. In one recent study, giving thyroid medication to women in this category reduced the risk of preterm birth by 70%.[9] The study authors noted that "women who are positive for thyroid antibodies before pregnancy may have subtle preexisting thyroid dysfunction that could possibly worsen during pregnancy." Even though someone may initially have normal hormone levels, the higher risk of complications may arise because the thyroid can't keep up with the demands of pregnancy, making it easy for an individual to slip into hypothyroidism.

This raises an important point for anyone already taking medication for hypothyroidism: you'll likely need to increase the dose of your medication by 25–30% during early pregnancy.

As explained by Dr. Elizabeth Pearce, an endocrinologist and an expert on thyroid hormones in pregnancy, "A woman who is treated for hypothyroidism before she becomes pregnant, even if she's got perfectly controlled thyroid blood tests before she conceives, is likely going to need an increase in her thyroid hormone dose." The increased need for thyroid hormone starts at around 7 weeks, so "we typically recommend a woman starts a higher dose as soon as she knows she's pregnant and continues that with frequent monitoring until she delivers."

The recommended treatment for underactive thyroid during pregnancy is levothyroxine. This is the same as natural T4 and can be converted by the body to T3 as needed. Other treatments made with desiccated animal thyroid, such as Armour Thyroid, are not recommended during pregnancy because they contain too much T3 and not enough T4. Only T4 can effectively cross the placenta, so if you're relying on Armour Thyroid, the supply of active thyroid hormones to your baby may fall short.

Iodine for Thyroid Function

Although most thyroid disorders in developed countries are caused by autoimmunity, iodine deficiency can still be an issue in some cases. Pregnancy places significant demands on the thyroid to produce more hormones than usual, which increases the need for iodine.

Severe iodine deficiency is uncommon in most developed countries, but approximately one-third of pregnant women in the United States have a mild deficiency, which can reduce thyroid function.[10] For this reason, organizations such as the American Academy of Pediatrics, the Endocrine Society, and the American Thyroid Association advise all pregnant women to take a prenatal supplement that contains 150 micrograms of iodine.

If your prenatal doesn't contain a significant amount of iodine, you can likely fill the gap by using iodized table salt rather than natural sea salt and by including more dairy and fish in your diet.

Seaweed is another rich source, but the amount of iodine can be unpredictable, and certain varieties may even contain too much. Extremely large doses of iodine can be counterproductive, causing oxidative damage to thyroid cells.[11] To prevent this, government bodies in several countries advise pregnant women to eat seaweed no more than once a week.[12]

Some doctors go further and advise patients with thyroid antibodies to avoid all supplements containing iodine, but there is little data supporting that approach. Current research suggests that supplementing with low doses of iodine (up to 200 micrograms) can reduce thyroid antibodies in individuals with Hashimoto's.[13]

Key Points

- Ask your doctor to check your TSH level as soon as possible during pregnancy.

- If your TSH is over 2.5 mIU/L or your T4 is less than 7.5 pg/mL, ask your doctor to test for thyroid antibodies and discuss whether you should take levothyroxine (Synthroid).

- If your TSH is only slightly elevated but you have thyroid antibodies, thyroid medication may lower the risk of miscarriage and preterm birth.

- Check that your prenatal multivitamin contains 150 micrograms of iodine. If it doesn't, use iodized salt and eat fish or dairy regularly to meet your daily iodine needs.

Chapter 8

Iron and Anemia

PREGNANCY DRAMATICALLY INCREASES the need for iron, especially during the second and third trimesters. During this time, a mother's blood volume increases by 50%, and a vast number of new red blood cells are needed to carry oxygen to the placenta.[1] Producing all these new red blood cells requires a steady supply of iron because it is a key component of hemoglobin, the protein in red blood cells that carries oxygen. The net result is that iron needs triple during the second half of pregnancy.

Maintaining optimal iron levels during pregnancy has a range of downstream benefits, including less fatigue, better sleep, stronger resistance to infections, and lower odds of preterm birth.[2] Studies have also found that maintaining sufficient iron levels during pregnancy can have long-term benefits for your baby's brain development.[3]

Iron is likely important to brain health because it supports the production of neurotransmitters, which carry signals between neurons.[4] Iron also supports the production of myelin, the protective layer around each neuron. When the billions of neurons in a child's brain have more of this protective layer, they can more easily carry signals, which results in improved memory and cognitive performance.[5] The benefits of getting enough iron during pregnancy can be seen many years later. Specifically, children born with higher iron levels at birth show improved language development, memory, self-regulation, and fine-motor skills by age five.[6]

The most important time for getting enough iron appears to be the third trimester. This is not only an important phase of brain growth but also when a baby needs to build up their own iron stores.[7]

These stores are critical because breastmilk provides only a marginal amount of iron. The American Academy of Pediatrics recommends that all exclusively breastfed babies receive iron supplements starting at four months. If a baby is born with low iron stores, this supplementation would need to be started even sooner. Supplementing can be difficult in newborns, however, because not all babies willingly take the strong-tasting drops and some may experience tummy pain. A better solution is prevention: giving babies enough iron during pregnancy to last through the first months.

How Much Is Enough?

The recommended intake of iron during pregnancy is at least 27 milligrams per day. Most good-quality prenatals include close to this amount, which leads many people to assume that a deficiency will not be an issue. Yet the amount of iron one can get from a prenatal and a typical diet is clearly not enough for many women to achieve adequate levels, particularly later in pregnancy. Even in the first trimester, approximately half of women in the United States are deficient.[8] The only way to know for sure if you are getting enough iron is to test.

Assessing Iron Levels

The most common lab value used to assess iron status is ferritin, a protein that stores iron inside cells. During pregnancy, ferritin should be at least 30 ng/mL. A low value indicates a need for additional iron. If your ferritin is normal or high, your iron intake is probably adequate. However, it's still possible to have a deficiency if your ferritin is elevated for other reasons, such as infection, inflammation, or even the pregnancy itself.

According to Dr. Michael Auerbach, a hematologist who has specialized in diagnosing and treating iron-deficiency anemia for more than 45 years, the most accurate way to assess iron levels during pregnancy is to test your transferrin saturation percentage.[9] This figure reflects the proportion of iron-transport proteins in your blood that are actually carrying iron. A value of less than 20% indicates the need for additional iron.[10] For greatest accuracy, transferrin saturation should be tested in the morning after fasting overnight.

Although this more accurate and expensive test is not generally necessary, you might consider it if your ferritin level is normal yet you notice symptoms of anemia, such as fatigue, pale skin, weakness, rapid heartbeat, dizziness, restless legs at night, or unusual cravings for ice. Iron levels are typically assessed at your first prenatal visit and then again between 24 and 28 weeks; there is usually no need for earlier or more frequent testing unless you notice symptoms.

Choosing an Iron Supplement

If your iron levels are low, adding a separate iron supplement will likely improve your energy levels and your baby's iron stores. The key is choosing a supplement in the optimal form.

Iron supplements are notorious for causing digestive side effects. The cheapest and most common forms, such as ferrous fumarate and ferrous sulfate, are poorly absorbed and can often cause constipation or nausea. A better option is iron bisglycinate, which combines iron and the amino acid glycine. This version rarely causes side effects, and it can effectively raise iron levels at a lower dose than standard forms.[11] In one randomized trial, a dose of 25 milligrams per day of iron bisglycinate was as effective as 50 milligrams of standard iron supplements, without the negative side effects.[12]

Another good supplement form is heme iron polypeptide, sold under the brand name Proferrin or Feosol Bifera. Derived from animal sources, it consists of iron bound to part of the hemoglobin protein and is much more readily absorbed than standard forms of iron, without the side effects. This form of heme iron also appears to raise ferritin levels even more effectively than iron bisglycinate. A typical dose is 20–30 milligrams per day.

Focusing on iron-rich foods may also help, although only to a limited extent. The best food sources are red meats such as beef and lamb, but even these foods contain only 5 milligrams of iron in a six-ounce serving, so it is difficult to meet daily iron needs through food alone. Beans and vegetables also contain some iron, but this form is very poorly absorbed, even with the help of vitamin C, so vegetarians and vegans usually need higher dose supplements.

After your baby is born, it's best to continue your iron supplement for at least the first month, to make up for blood loss and replenish your iron stores. This can have significant benefits for your mood and energy levels, with studies finding a clear link between higher iron levels in the month after delivery and a lower chance of developing postpartum depression.[13] One study randomly assigned women to an iron supplement or placebo starting one week after delivery and then assessed for postpartum depression after six weeks.[14] Those in the group taking iron were much less likely to develop signs of depression and saw a faster improvement than those in the placebo group. Somewhat surprisingly, taking an iron supplement during pregnancy doesn't appear to have as much impact on postpartum depression. It is iron intake in the month after delivery that matters most.[15]

Key Points

- Getting enough iron during pregnancy can help prevent anemia, reduce fatigue, boost immunity, and support your baby's brain development.

- The recommended intake of iron during pregnancy is 27 milligrams per day, but increasing this dose to at least 40 milligrams in the second half of pregnancy may be even better.

- Doctors typically assess iron status by measuring serum ferritin, which should be above 30 ng/mL.

- If your iron is low, consider supplementing with an additional 20–30 milligrams of iron bisglycinate or heme iron polypeptide. These forms are more effective and cause fewer side effects than standard iron supplements.

Chapter 9

Prenatal Testing

I N 1997, Dr. Dennis Lo and his colleagues at the University of Oxford made the startling discovery that during pregnancy, pieces of the baby's DNA can be detected in the maternal bloodstream.[1] This finding suggested it may one day be possible to assess whether the baby has a genetic condition simply by taking a sample of the mother's blood, bypassing invasive testing procedures such as amniocentesis. By 2011, this testing became a reality and quickly revolutionized prenatal screening for genetic disorders such as Down syndrome. Today, with a blood test drawn at around 10 weeks, a laboratory can screen for a range of genetic disorders.

This method, known as noninvasive prenatal testing, or NIPT for short, is now recommended as the default screening method in many countries. It is currently performed in over one-third of pregnancies in the United States, where guidelines recommend that NIPT be offered to all pregnant women. The test is less likely to be worthwhile if both partners are younger than 35 because in that situation, the chance of the baby having a genetic abnormality is very low. Even so, the only downside of having NIPT testing is the cost and potential for further unnecessary testing. For this reason, many couples decide to go ahead with the test even if they are considered low risk.

Before Dr. Lo's discovery, the odds of a baby having a serious genetic disorder were estimated by the combination of ultrasound measurements at 12 weeks and the presence of a specific protein in the blood. This old-fashioned screening method could identify 80–85% of cases of Down syndrome and several other conditions caused by an extra copy of a chromosome, with a 5% false positive rate.

NIPT testing is much more accurate, identifying these conditions more than 99% of the time and with fewer false positives, at least for the most common genetic conditions. A clear NIPT test is very reassuring and typically eliminates the need for amnio or chorionic villus sampling (CVS) unless an abnormality is seen on an ultrasound.

The problem with NIPT is that as companies have expanded testing beyond the most common genetic conditions (to detect abnormalities in sex chromosomes as well as small deletions or duplications), the number of false positives has increased dramatically.

The proportion of false positives in any given test is directly related to how rare a condition is. Even if a test has 99.9% specificity, meaning that it correctly identifies negative cases 99.9% of the time, that still represents 1,000 positive cases for every million people tested. If the condition is very rare and only occurs in 1 out of a million people, the test will have 999 false positives for every true positive. In short, the more uncommon a condition is, the more likely it is that a positive result is wrong.

A more meaningful way to assess the significance of a positive test is called the positive predictive value, which refers to the percentage chance that a positive result is a true positive. This value depends on both the accuracy of the test and how rare the condition is.

Most companies don't report this value for their tests, but a 2023 study found that the positive predictive value of NIPT testing for trisomy 21, trisomy 18, and trisomy 13 was between 80 and 100%, meaning that most positive tests are accurate.[2] For sex chromosome abnormalities, the value was 68%, and for other rare abnormalities it was just 25%, meaning that three quarters of positive results are incorrect. Other recent studies have found that only 50% of positive results for sex chromosome abnormalities are correct, even when a test is marketed as having 99.9% accuracy.[3]

This data highlights the fact that NIPT results should not be considered diagnostic, particularly for rare conditions. A positive result merely suggests the need for further testing, which your doctor can guide you through. You can also choose to consult a genetic counselor for more specific advice on next steps. Genetic counselors typically have master's degrees in genetics and so are well versed in interpreting and following up on NIPT results.

The high rate of false positives for rare conditions also calls into question whether it's worth paying more for newer and more costly "expanded" versions of NIPT tests that look for rare genetic changes called microdeletions, along with other uncommon abnormalities. The argument in favor of such testing is that it can catch genetic abnormalities associated with small deletions, such as DiGeorge syndrome. This condition, which occurs in approximately 1 in every 4,000 births, is one of the major causes of genetic heart defects and intellectual disabilities. It can be detected by expanded NIPT testing but not the conventional form of NIPT.

The argument against testing for microdeletions and other rare conditions is that it can be more expensive and most positive cases will be false positives, causing unnecessary anxiety and further testing.[4] In the case of DiGeorge syndrome, for example, approximately 82% of results flagged as "high risk" are false positives, with further testing indicating that the baby is perfectly healthy.[5]

If you do get a positive or "high risk" result from NIPT testing, the next step is usually a detailed ultrasound to see if any structural abnormalities are present. If the ultrasound is normal, the chance that a positive NIPT result is accurate drops to around 60%, depending on the condition.[6] From there, your doctor or genetic counselor can help you decide whether to have an amniocentesis, typically performed between 14 and 20 weeks of pregnancy, or CVS, performed between 10 and 13 weeks.

Although there can be a slightly longer wait for amniocentesis, experts often prefer that approach if you have already reached 12 or 13 weeks, as it can be more accurate for certain conditions. Both NIPT and CVS measure DNA that originates from cells of the placenta, whereas amniocentesis measures the baby's DNA floating in the amniotic fluid.

The genetic makeup of the placenta usually matches the DNA of the baby, but not always. Studies have found that when the placenta has a combination of normal and abnormal cells (a situation known as mosaicism), CVS and NIPT testing can be unreliable predictors of the baby's genetic status, whereas amniocentesis is more accurate.[7] This is more of a concern for some genetic conditions than for others. For Down syndrome, CVS is considered very accurate, but studies have found that CVS has greater rates of false positives for trisomy 18 and trisomy 13 because the abnormality can be confined to cells of the placenta.[8] For this reason, amniocentesis is typically the best option for a definitive answer. Although any procedure during pregnancy can be daunting, the most recent studies show that amniocentesis is very safe. The risk of miscarriage associated with the procedure is typically quoted as 1%, but the latest data shows that it is now even lower, at 0.12%.[9]

NIPT Testing with a PGT-Tested Embryo

If you're pregnant with an embryo that was already tested for chromosomal abnormalities by preimplantation genetic testing (PGT) during the IVF process, the odds of the baby having a genetic condition are vanishingly small. As a result, NIPT testing is much less useful and far more likely to return a false positive. One recent study found that if you receive a positive NIPT result with a PGT-tested embryo, the NIPT result will be a false positive an astonishing 92% of the time.[10]

Testing with both PGT and NIPT is largely redundant since they both test the DNA from the part of the embryo that becomes the placenta, and both methods look for abnormalities involving additional or missing copies of chromosomes. Although PGT testing is far from perfect, many obstetricians and genetic counselors advise that NIPT testing is unnecessary if your embryo was already genetically tested.

The main argument in favor of NIPT testing in this context is the ability to identify microdeletions, which are not tested with PGT. As mentioned earlier, the value of assessing for microdeletions is limited since these are rare and testing is therefore plagued by false positives. With that in mind, it's very much a personal decision whether testing is worthwhile. If you decide to go ahead with NIPT testing for added reassurance, remember that positive test results should be treated with great skepticism.

The Optimal Time for NIPT

Most NIPT companies advise that testing can be performed as soon as 10 weeks, although some doctors advise waiting until 11 or 12 weeks. Early testing provides more time to follow up on the results if needed, but it can also increase the odds of needing to repeat the test because of insufficient fetal DNA in your bloodstream. This problem occurs more often in women with a high BMI because the percentage of fetal DNA in the bloodstream is naturally lower. Age, autoimmune diseases, and the use of blood-thinning medication can also reduce the fetal fraction and increase the likelihood of having to retest. In these situations, it may be better to wait until 11 or 12 weeks.

If you're in the United States and NIPT is covered by your insurance, consider asking the testing company for a quote for the cash price, which might be significantly less than your insurance copay. In addition, if you go through insurance and still receive a large bill, you can often call the testing company to negotiate a lower out-of-pocket payment, typically around $250.

Surviving the Wait

Noninvasive prenatal testing has become a watershed event in pregnancy. Getting clear NIPT results and making it through the 12-week ultrasound is the point at which many couples can finally breathe a sigh of relief. Getting good news from both the ultrasound and NIPT is truly reassuring because at that point the chance of a serious problem is incredibly low and the miscarriage rate going forward is less than 1%.

If you've been through difficult times to reach this point, however, the wait for reassurance from NIPT results and ultrasounds can be agonizing. During this phase, it can help to learn some mindset techniques for coping with worries and uncertainty so you can worry less and enjoy more of your pregnancy. That's the subject of the next chapter.

Key Points

- Clear NIPT results are reassuring because this testing rarely misses genetic abnormalities.

- On the other hand, false positives are common, so a positive NIPT result merely suggests the need for further testing.

- Testing can be performed as soon as 10 weeks, but waiting until 11 or 12 weeks can reduce the chance of needing to repeat the test.

PART 3

Your Happiest, Healthiest Pregnancy

Chapter 10

Letting Go of Worry and Finding Joy

OUR BRAINS ARE hardwired to focus on potential threats and dangers, often allowing positive thoughts and experiences to slip by without notice. For millions of years, this hardwiring helped our ancestors survive by increasing focus on potential dangers and ensuring that negative experiences were etched into memory and avoided in the future. We're all descendants of the more stressed and worried members of ancient tribes—those who were more alert to potential dangers and therefore survived to pass along their genes. In the words of psychologist Rick Hanson, "the brain evolved a negativity bias that makes it like Velcro for bad experiences but Teflon for good ones." The result is that worrying and avoiding harm become our default way of thinking.

Although this bias was advantageous on the African savanna, in modern times it has much less value and can rob us of the joys of everyday life. This is particularly true in pregnancy, a time when worries about what can go wrong can easily overshadow what should be a happy time. You might feel a brief burst of excitement after the first positive pregnancy test but then find yourself in an anxious waiting game, scared to get excited until you make it over the next hurdle. Whether that's the first beta hCG blood test, hearing the heartbeat, getting a clear prenatal screening, or making it to viability, the goalposts often keep moving while you remain in suspense, focusing on the next milestone.

This torturous waiting game can be particularly overwhelming if you have a higher-risk pregnancy or experience with miscarriage or longstanding infertility, but it's also a universal pattern that unites all future parents with a tendency to worry. This response is simply the natural result of millions of years of evolution, creating a brain that focuses on past negative events and potential dangers while ignoring the good in the present moment.

This issue is all too familiar to me. With our surrogate's second pregnancy, after we lost an earlier pregnancy and had multiple failed embryo transfers, the fear of something going wrong always lurked just below the surface. Each time I started to feel a bit more confident that things were going well, the anxiety was restored by new issues, including low and slow-rising hCG numbers, then heavy bleeding at 12 weeks and difficulty finding a heartbeat on the ultrasound, then signs that we might be facing a very early preterm birth.

In the end, luck was on our side. After nine months of continual worry and believing that the best outcome we could hope for was an early preemie with a long NICU stay, we finally got one lucky break after another and ended up with a healthy, full-term baby boy who was cleared to go home after just a few days.

All that time spent imagining the worst made me even more grateful for his safe arrival. But if I could go back and change anything, it would be to give my past self some strategies to manage the negative thoughts and worry so I could enjoy what should have been a happy and exciting time. I wish I could have gone into ultrasounds looking forward to seeing a glimpse of my growing baby rather than terrified of more bad news.

That's the goal of this chapter: to arm you with evidence-based techniques for managing the anxieties that naturally crop up during pregnancy and to give you the chance to experience all the happy moments you can.

Letting in Joy

The first strategy focuses on elevating your default mental state and shifting your focus from worry to joy, so you can become more resilient and better prepared to face any challenges that may arise.

Psychologists have spent decades working on the problem of our natural bias toward negative thoughts and anxiety. They've shown that this state isn't inevitable or permanent: it's possible to rewire your brain so your default thought processes and feelings involve more joy and less worry, regardless of the circumstances. Importantly, this isn't about denying or ignoring every negative thought but rather recognizing that, although inevitable, these thoughts shouldn't keep you from noticing and experiencing the good moments.

One of the leading psychologists in this area is Dr. Rick Hanson, author of *Hardwiring Happiness, Resilient,* and other books on the science of positive psychology. Dr. Hanson's central thesis is that by taking in and fully immersing ourselves in everyday positive thoughts and experiences—no matter how small—we can change the brain's bias from negative to positive. Doing this can help you rein in anxious thoughts and allow you to live through times of uncertainty with much more peace and calm. In Dr. Hanson's words, "You're not looking at the world through rose-tinted glasses, but rather correcting your brain's tendency to look at it through smog-tinted ones."

One of the underlying principles of this philosophy is that our daily thought patterns can change the brain at a structural level. Everything we think and feel activates a specific electrical pathway in the brain. The more often a specific pathway is activated, the stronger the pathway becomes, like a trail in the woods that, over time and with more and more use, becomes wider, clearer, and easier to travel. As Dr. Hanson explains:

The brain takes its shape from what the mind rests upon. If you keep resting your mind on self-criticism, worries, grumbling about others, hurts, and stress, then your brain will be shaped into greater reactivity, vulnerability to anxiety and depressed mood, a narrow focus on threats and losses, and inclinations toward anger, sadness, and guilt. On the other hand, if you keep resting your mind on good events and conditions (someone was nice to you, there's a roof over your head), pleasant feelings, the things you do get done, physical pleasures, and your good intentions and qualities, then over time your brain will take a different shape, one with strength and resilience hardwired into it.

In short, your thoughts are shaped by a physical system that, like a muscle, gets stronger the more you exercise it. The specific exercise Dr. Hanson favors is called "taking in the good," which involves pausing to fully absorb and internalize positive experiences each day. Doing so activates a positive mental state that is then more likely to become etched in your brain as a default setting.

This positive experience could be anything happening in the present moment, or a happy thought or memory. To use a term coined by author Cyndie Spiegel, it's a choice to notice and appreciate the "microjoys" in everyday life. A microjoy could be as simple as noticing the feeling of being comfortable and cozy at home, appreciating something beautiful outside the window, being grateful for someone in your life, enjoying a favorite food, or anything big or small that makes you feel peaceful, grateful, happy, or cared for. The key is to stay with the experience long enough to let it fill your mind and flow through your body, perhaps visualizing the positive feeling as bringing warmth, beams of light, golden dust, or a protective bubble surrounding and protecting you. You can then draw on this feeling when you need to in order to lift you out of moments of worry.

This requires deliberate practice at first. You may have to consciously look for chances to let in good experiences. Over time, however, it becomes second nature. Your brain's default mode shifts toward noticing and appreciating the little things that bring you happiness. In effect, you're raising your default happiness set point—a concept backed by decades of research. When you later encounter stressful situations or difficult times, it will be easier to calm yourself and return to a better mental state.

Shutting Off the Stress Response

In moments of major stress or anxiety, focusing on the good can be a challenge and may not be enough to pull you out of the depths. In such times, it helps to understand how anxious thoughts can create a mental and physical stress response that can snowball and what steps you can take to escape this downward spiral.

The primitive part of your brain that lights up in response to stress is not very skilled at distinguishing between true dangers and everyday worries. It can easily overreact, triggering pathways designed for survival in dangerous situations and flooding your body with adrenalin and other stress hormones. This is known as the "fight-or-flight" response. The hormones and neurotransmitters that are released when you're stressed can often magnify worries and stop you from thinking clearly, allowing the stress and worry to build on itself.

If you find yourself feeling anxious before an ultrasound or after googling your latest pregnancy worry in the middle of the night, the first step is to get out of fight-or-flight mode and into a state of calm. To do so, the primitive part of your brain needs to be told that you're safe and everything will be okay. This message can be conveyed through your conscious thoughts or by using breathing exercises and other physical strategies that send signals from the body to the brain to trigger the relaxation response.

Activating the Relaxation Response

Just as the primitive part of the brain can be activated by signs of danger, which triggers the release of adrenalin, another system in the brain acts to turn off this response when the threat has passed. Known as the parasympathetic nervous system, it's a network of neural pathways that extends from the brain to other parts of the body. It constantly monitors and regulates heart rate, breathing pattern, and muscle tension.

There are many ways to activate the relaxation response, but one of the most effective is breathing as if you're already calm. By mimicking the slow, deep breathing pattern we normally follow when we're relaxed, we can shut down the release of adrenalin and other stress hormones and shift our brain and body into a more peaceful state.

Studies have found that consciously regulating your breathing can ease stress and anxiety even more effectively than long sessions of mindfulness meditation.[1] One of the studies demonstrating this, led by researchers at Stanford University, compared mindfulness meditation to five-minute breathing exercises such as box breathing and prolonged exhalation.[2]

The general principle of box breathing is to repeat cycles of slow breaths, with equal-length inhalations and exhalations—for example, inhaling for a count of four, holding for four, exhaling for four, then holding for four. Prolonged exhalation is a similar exercise, but each exhale is longer than each inhale. One particular method is 4-7-8 breathing, where you breathe in for a count of four, hold for seven, then breathe out for a count of eight. Following this pattern for five minutes is one of the best ways to activate the relaxation response.

In the Stanford study, these breathing exercises produced significant improvements in mood and anxiety levels—much greater than those seen with mindfulness meditation. The improvements were also cumulative, with more pronounced benefits when the breathing exercises were practiced daily for a month.

Other researchers have also demonstrated that by regularly using slow breathing to activate the relaxation response, you can train your nervous system to stay more relaxed in the face of stress. As a result, you become more resilient and better able to cope with difficult situations.[3] One of the studies demonstrating this effect involved veterans from the Iraq and Afghanistan wars who struggled with PTSD. Researchers found that daily breathing exercises not only helped normalize their anxiety levels after just one week, but the veterans continued to experience the mental health benefits a full year later.[4]

You can use breathing exercises as part of your daily routine to lower your stress levels and boost your resilience. You can also call on this strategy whenever you're feeling anxious or worried. In moments of anxiety, activating the relaxation response with slow, deep breathing is a good first step that allows you to think more clearly. This makes it easier to apply the next strategy, which involves changing how you feel by rewiring your thought patterns.

You can also perform slow, deep breathing as part of other practices for stress relief, such as yoga and Pilates. Yoga is the original source of many approaches that use breath to trigger the relaxation response, and coupling yoga-based breathing practices with other elements of yoga likely has even greater benefits. Pilates is another practice that involves slow, controlled breathing patterns that can help you shift from a state of stress to a state of calm. Pilates has the added advantage of building core strength and stability, as discussed in more detail in Chapter 14.

Questioning Negative Thoughts

Another helpful strategy for managing pregnancy worries is to treat your thoughts with skepticism and consciously challenge them. Some examples are given in the following sections, but the general principle is that when we're anxious, our brains tend to distort the facts—magnifying the negative and minimizing the positive. But anxious thoughts are just that: thoughts. You don't have to accept them as accurate or valid. In a way, your anxiety is like an overprotective friend, trying to keep you safe. You don't have to accept everything that friend says as true.

This concept of examining your thoughts and questioning their validity goes hand in hand with the proven technique of postponing worry: setting aside a short time later in the day to think about what's troubling you. When an anxious thought comes up, you simply let it go, noting that you can think about it later during your scheduled worry time. During that time, various strategies can help you move forward from what may be troubling you, including thinking about whether you have any power to alter the outcome. If so, you can plan active steps to take. If not, you can remind yourself that the matter is out of your hands and worrying won't help.

Another strategy is to postpone worrying until you have a legitimate reason to be concerned. You can diffuse anxious thoughts by acknowledging that, in the present moment, you have every reason to believe this pregnancy is going well and your baby will be healthy. If something changes in the future and you have a reason to be concerned, you can give yourself permission to worry then. But right now, when all signs are positive, there is no reason to worry.

A third strategy is to challenge your thoughts about the specific issue you're worried about, considering all the evidence in your favor and reassuring yourself that the odds are on your side. Doing so can help you gain a more balanced perspective and alleviate some of the anxiety surrounding the situation.

Concerns about external factors impacting your baby's health

One of the most common anxieties during pregnancy is worrying that some external factor beyond your control could cause harm to your unborn baby. This can include concerns about exposure to cigarette smoke, wildfires, chemicals, an unexpected illness, or a medication you need to take. In these situations, it can be helpful to remember two things. First, the uterus is a very protective environment that has evolved over thousands of years to keep babies safe from harm. Second, babies are incredibly resilient and can withstand more than we might expect. Thousands of pregnancies involve daily exposure to all manner of different hazards, and the vast majority of these babies are nevertheless born perfectly healthy.

In addition, all the positive steps you're taking to optimize your health will go a long way toward protecting your baby. The one negative factor you may be worried about will likely have much less impact than the thousand other positive efforts you are making.

When it comes to exposure to chemicals, pollution, and medications, for example, your supplement regime and healthy diet will make a big difference, protecting against potential harm by supporting your liver's ability to detoxify. This is particularly true of B vitamins and choline, which play a key role in breaking down chemicals through liver detoxification pathways. In addition, simply because you're doing your best to minimize exposure to chemicals when you can (as will be covered in Chapter 13), your overall level of exposure is likely much lower than average. This leaves your detoxification processes with plenty of capacity to handle the sources beyond your control.

In the case of infections and other external forces that can trigger inflammation, supplements such as omega-3 fats and vitamin D can reduce the potential harm by regulating the immune system. As just one example, studies have shown that the pregnancy complications that can arise following a severe COVID infection are much less likely to occur in women with adequate vitamin D levels.[5] The mechanism for this isn't fully understood, but it appears that vitamin D has protective effects on blood vessels in the placenta, while also helping prevent inflammation. We saw in earlier chapters that vitamin D and omega-3 fats can also help prevent many other consequences of infection and inflammation, including preeclampsia and preterm birth.

In short, by ensuring that you get enough of the critical nutrients your body needs during pregnancy, you're creating a protective force field around your baby. If you get sick or have moments of worry about other factors beyond your control, think about everything you're doing right to support your health and the fact that you're doing your best to create the most protective environment possible.

Concerns about pregnancy loss or complications

Another common source of worry is the possibility of pregnancy loss—a concern that may be heightened if you have experienced losses in the past or traveled a long, difficult path to pregnancy. This background can trigger self-protective thought patterns, including feeling detached from the pregnancy and being scared to get excited, panicking about daily fluctuations in pregnancy symptoms, and wanting constant reassurance that you're still pregnant.

Often these thoughts are coupled with the sense that something must be wrong with you for feeling this way instead of being able to celebrate where you are in this moment.

The reality is that worrying is perfectly normal, especially after experiencing problems in earlier pregnancies. Everything you're thinking and feeling is a reasonable response to what you've been through and simply a matter of self-preservation. Yet the fact that your anxiety is perfectly justified doesn't mean you're at its mercy. You can let go of the thoughts and worries that aren't serving you without sacrificing the protective shell you've built up to guard against possible disappointment.

One way to do this is by focusing on the here and now instead of ruminating on what's happened in the past or trying to look too far ahead into the future. This could involve staying busy and giving your attention to other positive things in your life as much as you can. Other strategies include simply taking your pregnancy day by day and reminding yourself that right now, in this present moment, you're pregnant, your baby is growing, and all signs are positive.

It's normal to want as much reassurance as possible during this time, and many women resort to using home pregnancy tests on a daily basis with the hope that seeing the line grow darker will ease their worries. Frequent home testing can be a double-edged sword, however, because these tests aren't designed to accurately measure the amount of hCG being produced. Instead, they aim to measure whether it's above a certain threshold. The darkness of the line can change from day to day for reasons that have nothing to do with the viability of your pregnancy, including the amount of water you drank the day before.

If you need confirmation that hCG is steadily increasing, it's better to ask for blood testing, if possible. If this testing shows that hCG has reached at least 100 mIU/ml by approximately two weeks after conception, and if the value is also doubling within 48 hours, the chance of miscarriage drops to less than 15%.[6] This is a more accurate tool to assess viability than monitoring with home pregnancy tests.

You can also reassure yourself that the odds are on your side. Our brain's natural negativity bias often clouds our thinking and can create the impression that a bad outcome is more likely than it actually is. When you actually look at the data, it is often more reassuring than you would expect.

In the case of bleeding during pregnancy, for example, it's natural to imagine the worst, but studies have found that when bleeding occurs between 7 and 11 weeks, after a heartbeat has been detected, there's over a 90% chance that everything will be fine.[7]

In the case of recurrent miscarriage, it's human nature to expect history to repeat itself. However, studies have found that even after three miscarriages in a row, the chance of a live birth in the next pregnancy is over 60%.[8] The odds remain promising in the pregnancy after that and the one after that. With each successive pregnancy, the total chance of a live birth continues to rise—by some estimates reaching over 95% across the next three pregnancies after three losses.[9] These statistics tell us that at some point, you'll likely have your rainbow baby. The past doesn't dictate the future.

In the case of pregnancy complications, it's also natural to be nervous about a recurrence. Yet most complications are less likely to happen again than you might expect. In this pregnancy, you are also much more informed, which gives you the opportunity to be more proactive and to focus on prevention and early detection. This is especially true for issues such as gestational diabetes and complications relating to the placenta, such as preeclampsia and preterm birth. In these cases, we have clear evidence-based strategies to shift the odds, as explained throughout this book. Chances are, this pregnancy will be better.

Finally, it's worth acknowledging your resilience. The fact that you've experienced difficulties in the past can be a source of strength, not just worry. When you're feeling anxious, remember that you're strong and resilient and have survived every challenge you've faced so far.

Key Points

- Counteract the brain's natural bias toward worry by taking in the good. Notice and fully absorb the small moments of joy in your day.

- Improve your resilience and ability to cope by using slow, deep breathing to activate the relaxation response.

- Question and challenge your negative thoughts rather than accepting them as true. You're doing everything you can to have a healthy pregnancy, and the odds are on your side.

Chapter 11

Managing Pregnancy Nausea

O NE OF THE most challenging obstacles to feeling good during early pregnancy, both mentally and physically, is nausea. This is a natural part of pregnancy that likely served an important evolutionary purpose, but that doesn't make it any easier to cope with. The past several years have brought fascinating new discoveries about what exactly causes pregnancy nausea and why some people are more affected than others. Hopefully, these discoveries will soon lead to new treatment options, but in the meantime, several strategies and medications can often ease symptoms. It also helps to remember that this phase is only temporary; most people find that nausea lifts or disappears entirely by 14 weeks.

Unraveling the Cause

Although most women experience some degree of nausea during pregnancy, the severity and duration vary widely. Up to 10% of women experience a more severe form of nausea and vomiting throughout pregnancy, a condition known as hyperemesis gravidarum. One person unlucky enough to experience this was Dr. Marlena Fejzo, a women's health researcher who had such severe nausea and vomiting during her second pregnancy that she became too weak to function. Troubled by the lack of research into severe pregnancy nausea, not to mention the dismissive response of her doctor, she fought for government funding to try to find the underlying cause. But her grant applications were met with little enthusiasm. This was no great surprise because the issue of pregnancy nausea has been neglected for decades. It has received barely any investment in research, even though it can be mentally and physically debilitating for thousands of women every year.

Unable to get sufficient funding for her own data collection, Dr. Fejzo approached the genetic testing company 23andMe, asking to mine their data set from thousands of individuals with the hope of finding clues as to what genes may be different in those with severe nausea. Before long, she found the link she was looking for: women with hyperemesis gravidarum were more likely to have specific variations in and around a gene encoding the hormone GDF-15, which stands for growth differentiation factor 15.[1]

This hormone is produced throughout the body in response to cellular stresses, including toxins, infections, and intense exercise. If you've ever felt sick after a strenuous workout, you can thank GDF-15. During pregnancy, it's produced in large amounts by the placenta, eventually reaching more than 200 times the normal level.[2] GDF-15 works by binding to receptors in the brain, causing nausea, vomiting, and food aversions. It may also suppress the immune system and play a role in insulin function.

The dramatic increase in GDF-15 production during pregnancy may have evolved as a mechanism to discourage consumption of potentially harmful foods during the first trimester, when the fetus is most vulnerable. The hormone may also regulate the immune system, orchestrating the changes to the immune system that are needed to sustain a healthy pregnancy. Another theory is that the placenta produces GDF-15 to increase insulin production. This would make up for other pregnancy hormones that compromise insulin function.[3] Whatever the mechanism, there was likely a powerful evolutionary reason for the placenta to start producing vast amounts of this hormone in early pregnancy.

After seeing the link between GDF-15 and pregnancy nausea, Dr. Fejzo went on to investigate the hormone in greater detail. Thanks to her groundbreaking research, it's now becoming clear that GDF-15 is one of the main factors driving the wide variability between women when it comes to the severity of nausea and vomiting during pregnancy.[4]

Interestingly, it's not just levels of GDF-15 during pregnancy that matter—it's also our individual sensitivity. If you had higher levels of GDF-15 before pregnancy, you may be much less sensitive and less likely to feel sick than someone who naturally had lower levels. That's because your brain can eventually become desensitized to signaling from GDF-15, so that it no longer causes symptoms. Dr. Fejzo and an international team demonstrated this phenomenon by showing that women with thalassemia, a blood disorder that chronically elevates

GDF-15, don't experience nausea during pregnancy.[5] "It completely obliterated all the nausea. They pretty much have next to zero symptoms in their pregnancies," said Dr. Stephen O'Rahilly, an endocrinologist at the University of Cambridge who was involved in the research. On the other hand, genetic variants associated with hyperemesis gravidarum cause much lower levels of GDF-15 before pregnancy, making women more sensitive to it when they are pregnant.[6]

How we use this new understanding to manage nausea in the real world is the big question. Given that this research is in its infancy, little guidance exists on how we can take advantage of the new discoveries to lessen symptoms. Even so, we can look for clues in prior research on GDF-15 that has been done outside the pregnancy context.

The first strategy suggested by that research is to start taking iron and B vitamins before you notice any nausea symptoms and to try to continue with supplements and a protein-rich diet once nausea starts, to the extent you can. Nutrient deficiencies can raise GDF-15 and make nausea worse, creating a vicious cycle. The particular nutrients that seem to have most impact are iron, thiamin, and amino acids.[7]

As mentioned in Chapter 1, standard iron supplements can temporarily exacerbate nausea, but supplements that contain heme iron polypeptide (such as Bifera) are much better tolerated. If you're able to continue taking this supplement, at least some days, that will help you avoid an exacerbation of nausea from iron deficiency.

Thiamin can have a significant impact as well. This B vitamin is quickly depleted if you're vomiting or unable to eat well, and a lack of thiamin will likely worsen nausea.[8] On the other hand, studies have reported a significant drop in GDF-15 after treating thiamin deficiency, which indicates that increasing thiamin intake through food or supplements may help ease symptoms.[9] The best food sources of thiamin are typically legumes, including peanuts, chickpeas, green peas, and black and navy beans. Pork, salmon, and oats are also good sources. If you're very sick and unable to eat much, additional thiamin supplementation may be helpful. Official guidelines recommend weekly thiamin injections or IV infusions for those hospitalized with hyperemesis gravidarum.

Animal studies also indicate that specific amino acid deficiencies can have an impact. It appears that a diet low in the amino acid lysine can increase GDF-15 and therefore nausea.[10] The best sources of lysine are soybeans, chicken, lentils, beef, eggs, and yogurt. If you're having trouble with these foods, consider trying a smoothie made with whey protein or pea protein powder, both of which are high in lysine.

The final—and probably most important—way we can influence GDF-15 levels is by maintaining steady blood sugar levels. GDF-15 is raised by the sudden spikes in blood glucose that occur after eating refined carbohydrates.[11] It also stays higher in those with poor insulin function and high fasting glucose levels. By keeping blood sugar under control, it may be possible to significantly lessen nausea. This creates a challenge if bread and crackers are the only foods you can tolerate, since these foods cause exaggerated spikes and crashes in blood sugar levels. To the extent that you can, try combining refined starches with a source of protein or fiber to slow down the release of glucose. That could mean adding a few nuts or carrot sticks to meals or snacks. Eating smaller amounts more often and walking after meals will also lessen blood sugar spikes.

These strategies can potentially reduce the severity of symptoms by reducing GDF-15 levels, but nausea may remain a problem for at least part of your pregnancy. The worst phase is usually around 8–9 weeks; most women feel much better by 14–16 weeks. In the intervening time, it's a matter of making it through each day in whatever way you can.

One of the best tools we have for managing pregnancy nausea is medication, and you shouldn't feel guilty if you need to go down that path. The starting option is a combination of vitamin B6 and an antihistamine such as Unisom or Benadryl. As mentioned in Chapter 1, the combination of B6 and Unisom corresponds exactly to the common prescription medication Diclegis. It's considered very safe to take during pregnancy, as is the prescription medication Zofran.[12]

Other strategies that may help include:

- eating a small amount every one to two hours to avoid an empty stomach;
- eating dry breakfast cereals (with minimal sugar) that are fortified with vitamins to provide a source of nutrients if you can't tolerate prenatal vitamins;
- drinking water in small amounts throughout the day but not during meals;
- drinking water with electrolytes to maintain better hydration;

- experimenting with still, sparkling, cold, and flavored waters to find what you can tolerate best.

For additional resources and support, see hyperemesis.org.

Is Lack of Nausea Bad Sign?

Some evidence indicates that early nausea is associated with a lower chance of miscarriage, likely because it reflects a strong and healthy placenta that's producing more hormones.[13] But it's also common to have a perfectly healthy pregnancy without feeling sick at all. Up to a quarter of women who go on to have a live birth don't experience any nausea or vomiting.[14]

If you don't yet notice any nausea or other pregnancy symptoms, or if your nausea comes and goes, don't let that worry you. Your brain could simply be less sensitive to the signal from GDF-15 that creates the feeling of nausea. It's also normal for symptoms to ebb and flow. If you feel less nausea on some days, there is most likely no cause for concern. Just seize the chance to take some vitamins and eat more nutritious food while you can.

Key Points

- Nausea is caused in large part by the brain's response to GDF-15, a hormone produced by the placenta.
- The most effective ways to lessen nausea include:
- staying well-hydrated and eating higher protein and nutrient-dense foods when you can;
- maintaining steady blood sugar levels and avoiding spikes from large servings of refined carbohydrates;
- taking medication, such as a combination of vitamin B6 and Unisom.

Chapter 12

The Big Nutrition Controversies

I N THE WORLD of pregnancy health, few topics stir as much debate and scrutiny as decisions over caffeine, alcohol, and the list of foods to avoid. This chapter aims to cut through the noise with an unbiased look at the latest evidence so you can make your own informed decisions.

Caffeine

The issue of how strictly to limit caffeine during pregnancy has been hotly debated for decades and this is one of the few areas in which the official guidance is probably not quite cautious enough. That's because it doesn't take into account the latest research findings showing an impact on fetal growth.

The American College of Obstetricians and Gynecologists (ACOG) and the UK National Health Service advise that pregnant women can safely consume up to 200 milligrams of caffeine, equivalent to two small cups of coffee per day. This is based on studies from the 1990s and early 2000s, which reported that the chance of miscarriage and stillbirth only rises when caffeine intake is over 300 milligrams per day.[1]

The most recent data on this question is somewhat inconsistent, but it suggests greater caution. The chance of miscarriage may actually start to rise with lower levels of caffeine intake, around 100 milligrams per day.[2] Some have discounted this research by claiming that the link between morning sickness and coffee intake obscures the results. The argument is that women who have more nausea are naturally less likely to miscarry and also less likely to drink coffee. Although those points may be true, researchers have found that the link between caffeine and miscarriage is independent of nausea symptoms, so we can't discount the data so easily.[3]

Regardless of the controversy over miscarriage risks, other potential effects of caffeine need to be considered, particularly the impact on a baby's growth. In recent years, numerous studies have found a link between caffeine intake during pregnancy and smaller birth size, even at levels of caffeine consumption generally considered safe.[4]

This impact shows up in two ways. The first is an increase in the percentage of babies with fetal growth restriction or who are born small for their gestational age, meaning below the 10th percentile for weight. The link between this diagnosis and caffeine intake has been observed in more than 30 years of research, but it was typically associated with heavy caffeine intake.[5] More recently, researchers found that each 100 milligrams of caffeine per day is associated with a 13% increase in the odds of a baby being small for gestational age.[6] Although this data should give us pause, the reality is that these forms of growth restriction are still quite rare.

The effects of caffeine on growth may be more widespread, however, by causing more subtle impacts on growth that fall short of a formal diagnosis of growth restriction. Initial studies on this issue were somewhat reassuring, but they were based on recalling caffeine consumption later in pregnancy or a reduction in caffeine intake after 20 weeks. One of the studies often relied on to dispute the link between caffeine and impaired growth involved randomly assigning a group of pregnant women in Denmark to drink either decaf or regular coffee, without identifying which was which.[7] The study found little difference in birth size between the two groups. Yet this study suffered from many serious flaws, including the fact that it only started in the second half of pregnancy and that half the women ignored the study rules and drank other caffeinated coffee, in addition to the coffee they were given. As a result, the findings of this study are essentially meaningless.

In 2021, researchers at the National Institutes of Health (NIH) performed a much more rigorous study in more than 2,000 pregnant women at low risk for growth restriction, observing their caffeine intake at around 10–13 weeks by both self-reporting and by measuring caffeine metabolites in the blood.[8]

The researchers found that women with caffeine intake equivalent to at least half a cup of coffee a day had slightly smaller babies than those who didn't consume any caffeine. For women consuming even more caffeine, the impact on birth size was greater. Notably, the babies weren't smaller because of less body fat. Instead, they had a shorter length and smaller head circumference, suggesting an effect that goes beyond energy metabolism. The researchers noted that caffeine is believed to cause blood vessels in the uterus and placenta to constrict, which could potentially reduce the supply of nutrients to the baby.

In a follow-up study published in 2022, the NIH researchers found that this impact on length at birth persists into childhood, with height differences still apparent many years later, even at an intake of 150 milligrams of caffeine per day.

The height discrepancy actually increased as the children grew older, starting at a 0.7 cm difference in four-year-olds and progressing to a height reduction of 2.2 cm (almost one inch) in eight-year-olds who were exposed to higher caffeine levels during pregnancy. Whether this would have much impact on a child's life is questionable, but it shows that caffeine probably isn't as innocuous as many experts claim.

Ultimately, this is an issue where your own judgment and level of caution should guide you, but the safest approach is to switch to decaf or half-caf, or limit your intake to half a cup or one small cup of coffee per day, or two cups of tea. It's your usual daily intake that matters most, so an occasional large cup of coffee when you need it probably won't have much impact. The effect of caffeine may also be lessened by the other strategies in this book that promote blood flow through the placenta and reduce the odds of growth restriction. These include being physically active and taking vitamin D, omega-3 fatty acids, and low-dose aspirin.

Alcohol

The unequivocal recommendation of the CDC and many other government bodies is that pregnant women should abstain from alcohol entirely. This rigid approach has been questioned in recent years, with some doubts about whether it's supported by the evidence.

One of the voices proclaiming that total avoidance of alcohol is unnecessary is Emily Oster, author of *Expecting Better: Why the Conventional Pregnancy Wisdom Is Wrong—and What You Really Need to Know*. Oster's 2013 book makes the argument that "there is no good evidence that light drinking during pregnancy negatively impacts your baby."

Experts in this area take a very different view. One is Dr. Susan Hemingway (formerly Astley), a professor of epidemiology and pediatrics at the University of Washington and a specialist in fetal alcohol syndrome. Dr. Hemingway runs a clinic that has diagnosed fetal alcohol spectrum disorders in over 3,000 children, spanning more than 30 years. Her interpretation of the data is unequivocal: "As a pediatric epidemiologist, I conclude a drink a day is not safe." She notes that "1 out of every 14 children we have diagnosed with full blown fetal alcohol syndrome over the past 20 years had a reported exposure of just 1 drink per day."

On the other side of the debate, those who support moderate alcohol consumption in pregnancy often rely on a study in Denmark that investigated the link between alcohol consumption and measures of intelligence, behavior, and attention scores in children. The study found that up to eight drinks per week had no effect on those measures.[9] Yet it had one major flaw: the analysis stopped at preschool age.

The data from other studies, along with Dr. Hemingway's clinical experience, clearly show that negative impacts may emerge later in childhood. As she explains, "children exposed to and damaged by prenatal alcohol exposure do deceptively well in their preschool years. The full impact of their alcohol exposure will not be evident until their adolescent years."[10]

In Dr. Hemingway's data, which covers thousands of children assessed for fetal alcohol syndrome in her clinics, half of the children had normal developmental scores as preschoolers, but all had noticeable brain dysfunction by age 10. In addition, very few of the children with fetal alcohol syndrome had attention problems by age 5, but most developed them by the age of 10.

It's clear, then, that if we want to find out how low-level alcohol exposure during pregnancy is impacting brain function, we need to assess that function later in childhood rather than making decisions based on studies that stop at preschool age. Fortunately, that research has now been done, and we have much clearer answers than even a few years ago.

The most recent data convincingly shows that children exposed to even low levels of alcohol intake during pregnancy, on average 1 drink per week, are much more likely to have behavioral problems at 10 years old.[11] These behavioral problems include hyperactivity, difficulty with focus and attention, and increased aggression. Although some of the early studies reporting these trends could be criticized as failing to control for other factors that are more common in women who drink during pregnancy, such as smoking, that's not the case in the most recent studies.

A 2022 study in Canada, for instance, recruited more than 10,000 children, then carefully matched 200 of those children exposed to low levels of alcohol during pregnancy with 200 who were not exposed to any but who were otherwise very similar in terms of maternal education, family income, and several other variables. None of the children were exposed to smoking or drug use in pregnancy.[12]

The average alcohol intake in the exposed group was just one drink per week, and even this amount was found to be associated with increased aggression and other behavioral problems when the children were 10 years old. The researchers also performed MRIs and observed structural brain changes in the alcohol-exposed group that are known to be linked to behavioral problems. The researchers concluded, "From a policy perspective, our findings support the recommendations of the Centers for Disease Control and Prevention and the Society of Obstetricians and Gynaecologists of Canada, both of which recommend against any amount of alcohol consumption during pregnancy." Based on all the evidence available to us today, that is probably the best advice.

From a practical standpoint, if you decide to abstain completely from alcohol during pregnancy, you may wonder where the line should be drawn when it comes to alcoholic ingredients in cooking. Some worry about using vanilla extract, for instance, which can contain up to 35% alcohol. This is not really a concern since the amount used in a recipe is typically very small. On the other hand, it's probably advisable not to cook with wine or spirits as a main ingredient on a regular basis unless the dish will be cooked for several hours.

Although alcohol does evaporate during cooking, more remains behind than you might expect. According to the U.S.

Department of Agriculture, baked or simmered dishes that contain alcohol retain 40% of the original amount after 15 minutes of cooking and 25% after an hour. Good substitutes for wine in cooking include diluted red wine vinegar, chicken broth, and pomegranate or cranberry juice.

Preventing Foodborne Illness

Most of the well-known "food rules" during pregnancy are intended to avoid the foods with the highest risk of bacterial contamination—for good reason. The immune system undergoes major changes during pregnancy to prevent rejection of the placenta. This transformation also dials back immunity to infections, so pregnant women are much more likely to get sick from contaminated food. The most relevant type of food poisoning is caused by the bacteria *Listeria*. According to the CDC, pregnant women are ten times more likely to get sick from *Listeria* than the general population. This type of food poisoning also has much greater impact during pregnancy because the bacteria can cross the placenta and, in very rare cases, can cause pregnancy loss or health problems for the baby.

For many years, the standard advice has been to avoid foods that pose the highest risk for *Listeria*, including deli meats, soft cheeses, and any dairy products made from raw milk. Some people have suggested that this advice is outdated and that modern food-production methods have rendered these foods generally safe.

When we look at the FDA data, however, it's clear that *Listeria* is still being found exactly where we might expect: in soft cheeses such as Brie, Camembert, and queso fresco, and in precooked meats and deli meats. Several outbreaks have also been traced to small ice cream companies and bagged salads.

With any of these foods, the chance of a particular item containing *Listeria* is very small. In recent testing, only six out of more than 3,000 prepackaged deli meats were found to contain *Listeria*.[13] The odds of contamination were eight times higher for products sliced in-store and purchased from a deli counter, likely because of contaminated slicing equipment.[14]

Avoiding these higher-risk foods during pregnancy is akin to wearing a seat belt every time you drive—the chance of something bad happening is incredibly low, but it's still reasonable to take precautions.

When it comes to deli meats such as ham, turkey, salami, or sausages, the safest approach is to cook these foods until steaming hot. Frying ham or turkey in a small amount of oil before making a sandwich usually works well. The next best option is to choose packaged deli meats from large, reputable brands that are more likely to have careful quality-control procedures. You can also reduce the risk by purchasing these foods from a large store with fast turnover, so the package is fresh, and using items within several days of purchase.

Soft cheeses are another major culprit when it comes to *Listeria*. The FDA guidance is to avoid feta, Brie, Camembert, blue-veined cheeses, queso blanco, and queso fresco unless made with pasteurized milk. Unfortunately, pasteurization doesn't really solve the problem. Although the process sterilizes the milk, thereby eliminating the risk of *Listeria* originating from the milk itself, the bacteria is ubiquitous in the environment and is often introduced during further processing, either by humans or contaminated equipment. Because *Listeria* can grow quickly in soft cheeses at refrigerated temperatures, the risk is still relatively high. We know this from the many recent *Listeria* cases involving Brie and Camembert made with pasteurized milk. In recent years, the FDA has recalled more than twenty brands of these soft cheeses because of *Listeria* contamination in the manufacturing facility. As with deli meats, the safest approach is to eat only soft cheeses that have been thoroughly heated.

Another high-risk item is bagged lettuce and salad. Every year, there are several recalls for bagged salads, whether due to *Listeria* or *Salmonella*. These products pose a higher risk than a whole head of lettuce because any cut or damaged leaves allow bacteria to attach and grow exponentially, contaminating an entire batch. Researchers in England found that a small amount of juice released from cut or crushed lettuce leaves allowed *Salmonella* to grow 2,000-fold compared to a control sample. Studies have also found that it's difficult to remove bacteria from lettuce and other vegetables that have been precut. It's much safer to buy a whole head of lettuce and wash it thoroughly before use. Soaking leaves in diluted vinegar solution before rinsing is even more effective than washing with plain water.

Along with *Salmonella, E. coli* is another bacteria to watch for. Although it's most commonly found in raw and undercooked poultry, meat, and eggs, the FDA has also reported frequent outbreaks in alfalfa sprouts, cantaloupe, and bagged romaine lettuce, usually from contamination during farming. As such, these foods may not be worth the risk when safer options are readily available. It's also worth following the standard advice of ensuring that meat, seafood, and eggs are thoroughly cooked before serving. Fortunately, *Salmonella* and *E. coli* are less likely to impact your baby during pregnancy than *Listeria*, so it's a judgment call as to how careful you choose to be.

If you do get food poisoning at some point in your pregnancy, rest assured that you can most often conquer the illness within a few days, with no lasting impacts. If you experience ongoing symptoms such as headache, fever, muscle aches, and backaches, you can ask your doctor for a blood test for *Listeria*. If the test comes back positive, antibiotic treatment is often very effective at preventing later pregnancy complications.

Key Points

- Caffeine intake during pregnancy may slightly increase the odds of miscarriage and can impact a child's growth. The safest approach is to switch to decaf or half-caf or limit your intake to half a cup or one small cup of coffee per day, or two cups of tea. Occasional intake greater than this is unlikely to pose a problem.

- New research shows that even minor intake of alcohol in pregnancy can compromise children's brain development. This was not seen in earlier studies because the effects often become evident later in childhood.

- Traditional advice to avoid soft cheeses, deli meats, and bagged salads during pregnancy is grounded in science. The odds of getting sick are low, but these are the highest-risk foods, and some caution is warranted.

Chapter 13

Minimizing Toxins and Finding Balance

R EDUCING YOUR EXPOSURE to chemicals during pregnancy can have profound benefits for both you and your baby, including lowering the chance of preterm birth and protecting your baby's brain development. Yet with new headlines every week sounding the alarm about the dangers of everything from non-stick chemicals to pesticides to microplastics, it can be hard to know where to start. The key is to focus on the issues that have the most impact, rather than striving to eliminate every potential source of toxin exposure.

Our bodies have a remarkable ability to detoxify and withstand chemical insults. At any given moment, your liver is working hard to break down and help you excrete all manner of compounds. This include toxins created by your cells during normal metabolism as well as those you may be exposed to through the air you breathe, the food you eat, and the products you use on your skin. All are being continuously broken down and removed from your body.

Healthy foods, along with the vitamins and minerals found in your prenatal, strengthen your defenses further. The liver uses B vitamins, vitamin E, zinc, selenium, and choline in an elaborate chain of reactions to break down toxins. By taking a good-quality prenatal and the other supplements mentioned in earlier chapters, and by choosing nutrient-dense whole foods when you can, you're building up a defense system to help protect you and your baby from chemicals in the environment.

You can support this system further by reducing your exposure to toxins when it is easy to do so. This will lighten the burden on your liver and decrease the impact of chemicals that are harder to avoid. Simply lowering the overall dose is helpful because for many toxins, there is a threshold effect: small amounts have little to no impact on our health, while larger exposures have noticeable effects. That's because smaller amounts can be metabolized and excreted before they cause harm. In addition, for chemicals that cause negative impacts by interfering with hormone activity (so called "endocrine disruptors"), it's likely that our hormone systems can adapt and withstand minor disturbances. Problems may only occur when the total exposure level is enough to overwhelm the body's ability to regulate hormonal activity.

The goal, then, is to do what you can to choose safer products and reduce chemical exposure when it is easy to do so, then try not to worry about the matters beyond your control. This is a situation where the Pareto principle applies: you'll likely get most of the benefit from the first 20% of effort—focusing on making a few simple changes and replacing the products that matter most.

As this chapter explains, the chemicals that are most helpful to avoid during pregnancy fall into four general categories:

1. **Pesticides**, found in insect and weed killers and sprayed on crops
2. **Bisphenols**, found in hard plastic kitchenware and highly processed food
3. **Non-stick chemicals**, found in pots and pans and processed foods
4. **Phthalates**, found in processed food, fragranced items, and fabric softener

Reducing exposure to these compounds may require an initial investment to upgrade your cleaning products, skin care routine, and some of your kitchen items, but the benefits will continue long after your pregnancy—creating a safer and greener home for your little one to grow up in.

If you already took active steps to minimize toxin exposure while trying to conceive, many of the principles in this chapter will be familiar, and you're likely most of the way there. The same practical steps recommended in *It Starts with the Egg* apply during pregnancy, just with different benefits. Instead of protecting your egg quality and fertility, you'll be protecting your baby's development. There are, however, a few additional sources of chemical exposure that take on greater significance during pregnancy, such as pesticides and certain skin care ingredients.

The Problem with Pesticides

When it comes to creating a less toxic home during pregnancy, one of the highest priorities is tackling pesticides—all those chemicals used to control unwanted insects, weeds, or other living organisms. Pesticides are sprayed on crops, gardens, and pets as well as inside homes, often without much thought. But these compounds are, by their very nature, intended to be toxic. They're primarily toxic to the weeds, insects, and other pests they target, but when the concentration is high enough, they're also harmful to humans. A range of health problems, including an increased risk of asthma and certain cancers, have now been linked to the common pesticides used in homes and food production.[1]

When babies are exposed to these chemicals during critical windows of development, there is also a significant risk to brain development.[2] For more than a decade, the American Academy of Pediatrics (AAP) has been urging parents to reduce pesticide exposure during pregnancy and early childhood in order to protect brain development during this vulnerable time.[3]

We now have clear data showing that doing so is worthwhile, with recent studies reporting that minimizing pesticide exposure during pregnancy can have benefits that last throughout childhood, including improved cognitive function and a lower risk of neurodevelopmental disorders.[4] Much of this research has focused on the specific pesticide glyphosate, which is the active ingredient in the weed killer Roundup and the most heavily used pesticide in history. A recent study of pregnant women in Puerto Rico demonstrated that babies exposed to lower levels of glyphosate during pregnancy have improved language and cognitive scores at one and two years old.[5]

Practical Steps to Take

You can go a long way toward reducing your baby's exposure to chemicals such as glyphosate simply by choosing more organic foods, particularly for products made from wheat, oats, and corn.[6] Conventional producers typically spray these crops with glyphosate immediately before harvesting to dry the crops, which leads to very high levels on the final grain.[7] Lab tests commissioned by the Environmental Working Group recently found glyphosate in almost all products made with conventionally grown oats. Nearly three-quarters of the samples had glyphosate levels higher than what EWG scientists consider safe.[8] In comparison, none of the organic oats they tested contained glyphosate levels above this benchmark.

For fresh fruit and vegetables, there is less evidence that trace amounts of pesticide residues cause any harm. However, if budget permits and you live in an area where organic produce is available, it's reasonable to err on the side of caution and buy more organic foods when possible. This is more likely to be worthwhile for the fruits and vegetables known to carry higher levels of pesticide residues, namely:

- berries
- peaches
- pears
- peppers
- potatoes
- grapes
- apples
- spinach
- tomatoes
- kale

Peeling non-organic fruit and vegetables is also a good cautionary step, especially in the case of apples and pears. For berries and leafy greens, you can significantly reduce pesticide residues by soaking in a dilute baking soda solution. A recent study found that soaking fruit for 15 minutes in one teaspoon of baking soda and two cups of water can remove pesticides far more effectively than other washing methods.[9] It also helps to rely more heavily on fruits and vegetables that typically have low levels of pesticides, including:

- papaya
- honeydew
- pineapple
- onion
- cabbage
- asparagus
- mango
- kiwi
- avocado
- peas
- broccoli
- cauliflower

You may decide to go even further by choosing organic meats and dairy as well, and doing so is likely to have advantages, but here the balance between the potential health benefits versus higher cost is not as clear. Buying grass-fed or pasture-raised meat, butter, and eggs is likely a higher priority than buying organic because this will increase your intake of beneficial fatty acids and vitamin A.

Beyond food, it's also possible to dramatically reduce your exposure to pesticides by using better strategies to tackle weeds and insects in your home and garden. Rather than using Roundup or similar products in your garden, you can pull weeds by hand, use barrier cloths, mulch, and other plants, or let nature run a little more wild. To manage ants and other insects, bait stations are generally a safe option, allowing you to avoid chemical sprays that may be inhaled. For pets, it's best to use oral tablets or other natural methods of flea and tick control rather than topical treatments.

The Nontoxic Kitchen

The next culprit to focus on is Bisphenol-A, or BPA for short. Found in reusable hard plastics and can linings, this is one of the most well-known toxins that can disrupt the function of our hormones. Following years of heated controversy, many companies have phased out the use of this chemical, but it's still present in a variety of places, and many manufacturers are simply replacing BPA with closely related compounds that appear to act in much the same way.

Reducing exposure to these chemicals during pregnancy has a range of benefits, including protecting your baby's developing brain. Over the past fifteen years, numerous studies have reported that children exposed to higher levels of BPA during pregnancy and early childhood are more likely to have difficulties with behavioral and emotional regulation.[10] This is reflected in an increase in hyperactivity, aggression, anxiety, and learning problems.[11]

Now that fewer products on store shelves contain BPA, it's becoming easier to protect children from this threat, but you can make even more progress with a few swaps and changes to your routine. It's important to find some balance in this process, though. You don't have to replace everything or try to avoid BPA completely. Instead, the goal is to ensure that you don't have an unusually high level of exposure by avoiding the worst offenders.

By far the most useful step is eating more foods you prepare yourself at home from natural ingredients. Fast food and highly processed food can contain high levels of BPA due to contact with plastic equipment during processing. Another important step is swapping canned foods for alternatives in foil pouches or glass bottles, particularly for acidic items such as tomatoes.[12] Canned beans are less problematic, but it's still better to buy dried or frozen beans when you can. Otherwise, look for a brand labeled BPA-free. For canned fish such as salmon and sardines, the benefit to your baby of consuming the omega-3 fats during pregnancy likely outweighs the risks from the can lining. Even so, the best option is to rely on fresh or frozen fish, or foil pouches.

You can reduce your exposure to BPA even further by replacing reusable plastic food storage containers, travel coffee mugs, and other plastic items in your kitchen with stainless steel or glass. This is not something you have to do all at once, but it's most helpful for items that will be in contact with hot foods or liquids because heat causes more chemicals to leach from plastic.

For this reason, tea kettles and coffee makers with plastic internal parts are high priorities to upgrade. The safest way to make coffee is with a metal pour-over filter or a traditional French press made from stainless steel or glass, without plastic components.

As you go further down this path, it becomes clear that using some plastic in the kitchen is unavoidable. It's difficult to find high-performance blenders and water filters without plastic, for example. For these and other items, the key is to wash by hand in cold water and replace any container that is old and scratched. For blending hot soups and making baby food purees with hot ingredients, the best option is to use a stainless-steel immersion blender or a blender with a glass or stainless-steel container.

For food storage containers, it's helpful to replace any old or damaged plastic items with stainless steel or glass. When you do need to store food in plastic containers, look for high-density polyethylene (HDPE) or polypropylene, both of which are relatively safe.

Plastic food packaging and single-use water bottles typically don't contain BPA, but it's still better to choose glass bottles or purified tap water when you have the option. That's because bottled water may contain microplastics—tiny particles that are released as plastic breaks down. When ingested, they eventually make their way into various tissues in the body, including the placenta.[13] It's not yet clear what impact microplastics have during pregnancy, if any, but their presence weighs in favor of choosing filtered tap water over plastic bottled water when convenient. This is not a major concern, however, and staying hydrated likely matters far more than avoiding microplastics.

It's also worth reminding yourself that the goal isn't to completely avoid BPA and similar chemicals but rather to start reducing your overall exposure. This means making a few changes to items that make the most difference, such as avoiding canned tomatoes and plastic containers that will come in contact with hot foods or liquids. Just these small changes may be enough to make a significant difference, helping to support your baby's healthy brain development.

Safer Cookware

One last item to consider replacing in your kitchen is your non-stick pan. Research indicates that pregnant women with higher exposure to non-stick chemicals are more likely to have babies who are born premature or with a low birth weight.[14] Exposure to these chemicals during pregnancy also appears to impact the developing brain, resulting in lower cognitive scores, delayed language development, and increased odds of behavioral difficulties later in childhood.[15]

Non-stick pans pose the greatest problem when they become old and damaged or when heated to very high temperatures. Just replacing an old and damaged non-stick pan with a newer one and cooking at moderate temperatures makes a difference. Choosing a ceramic non-stick pan that is labeled "PFOA free" and "PTFE free" is also a vastly better choice than standard Teflon.

You can further reduce your exposure to non-stick chemicals by using this type of cookware only when needed and doing most of your cooking with even safer options. The best materials include cast iron, glass, and stainless steel. Silicone is also a generally safe material, although silicone baking trays and liners are best avoided because this material can leach chemicals called siloxanes at high temperatures.[16] Little is known about the long-term safety of siloxanes, so it's better to avoid unnecessary exposure.

For baking trays and sheet pans, once you're avoiding non-stick coatings, most other options will be made from aluminum. There is some controversy over this metal, but it's likely fairly safe since most aluminum we ingest is never absorbed into the body.[17] An even better strategy, though, is to use stainless steel sheet pans or glass baking dishes.

For specific product recommendations,
see itstartswiththebump.com/cookware.

Our Phthalate-Filled World

Many of the steps you can take to minimize exposure to BPA will have the added benefit of reducing your exposure to another group of chemicals known as phthalates. These chemicals are used to make fragrances last longer and to make fabric soft and flexible. They have a range of potential impacts during pregnancy, likely because they can disrupt testosterone function and thyroid hormones. As a result, a high level of phthalate exposure during pregnancy appears to contribute to genital malformations in baby boys.[18] Studies have also reported a link between phthalates and premature birth.[19] One possible explanation is that these chemicals increase inflammation, which raises the risk of earlier labor.[20] Dozens of studies have also reported negative impacts on behavior and cognitive function later in childhood, with greater rates of aggressive behavior, attention deficits, and language delay. [21]

Fortunately, governments have finally recognized the harms posed by these compounds and have started to limit their use. In many countries, specific phthalates are now banned in a variety of products, including food-handling equipment, toys, fragrances, and cosmetics.

These changes are clearly having an effect. Lab tests of thousands of individuals show that over the past ten years, there has been a steady decline in our exposure to phthalates.[22] This goes to show that change is possible, but it's still too soon to become complacent, and it's worth taking a few extra steps to reduce your exposure even further.

Practical Steps to Minimize Phthalates

As we saw with BPA, the one shift that has the greatest impact when it comes to phthalates is reducing your intake of highly processed food and fast food.[23] Boxed mac and cheese, for example, can have phthalate levels four times higher than a version you make yourself from natural cheese.[24] As explained by one researcher in the field, "there are so many steps to get to that boxed product, and every step along the way, there's usually plastic involved."[25] By preparing meals from scratch using fresh ingredients, it is possible to dramatically lower phthalate levels in just a few days.[26]

We also know that it's processing, not packaging, that matters most. In general, plastic food packaging is not a major concern.[27] The exception to this rule might be oil and acidic condiments because fats and acids can increase chemical leaching. It is worth buying these items in glass bottles, but for other items, there is typically no need to worry about plastic containers or bags.

Apart from processed food, the other major way we are exposed to phthalates is through fragranced items, including perfume, skin care products, air fresheners, and laundry products.[28] Phthalates are added to these products to help scents linger. They're also added to products such as fabric softener, nail polish, and hair styling products to give structure and flexibility. For this reason, it's helpful to simplify your routine and begin replacing products with versions labeled as phthalate-free or fragrance-free. Starting with your body lotion is a good step since it's applied over a larger surface area, which provides more opportunity for chemicals to be absorbed through the skin. For product recommendations, see itstartswiththe-bump.com/skincare.

How much further you choose to go in replacing your cosmetics and cleaning products is up to you, but every little bit helps. Additional items to consider replacing include PVC shower curtains and yoga mats. Look for a shower curtain made from nylon and a yoga mat labeled "PVC free" or "phthalate free." To replace fabric softener, vinegar and wool dryer balls are good alternatives.

Other Skincare Ingredients to Watch For

Parabens are commonly used preservatives typically found in lotions, sunscreens, and other personal care products. For many years it has been known that parabens disrupt hormones and fertility, but new research indicates that exposure to parabens during pregnancy may also compromise infant brain development.[29]

Triclosan is an antimicrobial chemical often found in antibacterial hand soap. It has now been recognized as a potent endocrine disruptor, causing disturbances to thyroid hormone levels during pregnancy.[30]

Chemical sunscreens can also act as hormone disruptors. The worst is oxybenzone, which is added to the majority of non-mineral sunscreens and has been found to lower testosterone levels, reduce pregnancy duration, and alter birth weights.[31] Safer sunscreen ingredients include zinc and titanium dioxide.

Retinols are vitamin A derivatives that are often added to antiaging skin care products. High doses can potentially interfere with fetal development and lead to birth defects. For this reason, pregnant women are typically advised to avoid products containing retinol and other similar derivatives such as Retin-A and retinoic acid.

Salicylic acid is a chemical exfoliant often included in acne treatments, but it can also be found in cleansers and moisturizers. Pregnant women are usually advised to avoid salicylic acid because it can be absorbed through the skin and has aspirin-like effects. Some doctors advise that up to 2% salicylic acid is safe to treat acne during pregnancy, but azelaic acid or topical antibiotics such as erythromycin and clindamycin are considered better options.[32]

Key Points

Reducing your exposure to chemicals during pregnancy has a range of benefits, including lowering the chance of preterm birth and protecting your baby's brain development.

You can make the most impact by:

- Minimizing the use of chemical weed killers and insect sprays
- Choosing more organic foods and preparing meals at home from fresh ingredients
- Replacing plastic kitchenware with glass or stainless steel
- Avoiding perfume, air freshener, and fabric softener
- Replacing scented products with fragrance-free versions

Chapter 14

Exercises for an Easier Pregnancy and Recovery

WOMEN ARE OFTEN told to avoid abdominal exercises during pregnancy, but this advice is likely overcautious and counterproductive. The data shows that developing a strong and stable core has a range of benefits. They include preventing back pain, shortening labor, minimizing tearing and other complications during delivery, and helping you recover more easily during the postpartum phase. The key is knowing which exercises to avoid and which ones have the greatest positive impact.

The Importance of Core Strength and Stability

More than 70% of women experience some back pain during pregnancy.[1] This is due to a combination of the increased load from a growing belly and hormonal changes that loosen ligaments and make the spine less stable. Studies show that having a strong core is the best way to prevent and reduce this pain.[2]

One of the most important core muscles for preventing back pain is the transversus abdominis, often referred to as the transverse ab or TVA, which wraps around your lower abdomen and acts as a corset or brace to stabilize the spine. Unlike other abdominal muscles, which move the spine in various directions, this deep core muscle is responsible for stabilization rather than movement. Other important core muscles include the obliques, which are located on the sides of your torso; the multifidus, which runs the length of the spine and stabilizes each vertebra; and the pelvic floor, which acts as a hammock to support the pelvic organs.

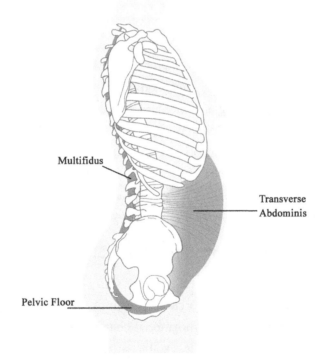

Figure 1. Essential muscles for core stability.

All these muscles work together to provide stability to your lower back. When functioning correctly, they should switch on and stabilize your core just before you move, bend, or lift a heavy object in order to minimize the load on your spine. If your core muscles are weak or don't activate when they should, the joints in your spine will have less support, and your lower back muscles can become sore and tense to compensate. On the other hand, when you strengthen your deep core muscles and learn to activate them automatically, your back becomes much more stable and less likely to cause you pain.

Developing good core strength also has many other benefits during pregnancy. As just one example, researchers have found that women who regularly perform Pilates or other exercises that activate the core tend to have a significantly shorter and easier labor.[3] In one of these studies, the average length of labor in a group of women following an exercise program was six and a half hours, compared to more than nine hours in the control group.[4] Exercises that activate the pelvic floor may also reduce the chance of significant tearing during delivery, lessen the chance of abdominal muscle separation, and help you recover more easily after delivery.[5]

Getting Started

If you're adding core exercises to your pregnancy routine for the first time, it can be helpful to start with guidance from a prenatal physical therapist or prenatal Pilates or yoga instructor. There are also many good online prenatal exercise programs developed by physical therapists and other experts. Another option is following the many free videos from physical therapists that are available online. (For examples see itstartswiththebump.com/core-stability). Regardless of which path you choose, the first and most important step is learning to activate the transverse ab muscle.

Transverse Ab Activation

To switch on this all-important muscle, start by lying on your back with knees bent and feet flat on the floor. Your lower back should be in a neutral position, not flattened into the floor. Place your fingertips on each hip bone and move them inward toward your midline by one to two inches. Inhale, then exhale through pursed lips, imagining you're drawing your hip bones together and gently sucking your lower abdomen toward your spine. You should feel the muscle harden slightly beneath your fingertips. This is your transversus abdominis.

You can also practice this activation when sitting and standing, using the same method. Once you learn how to turn on the muscle, the next step is to challenge the stability it provides by introducing movement of your arms or legs. One way to do this is with the bird dog, a popular exercise recommended by many prenatal physical therapists.

To perform this exercise, start on all fours, with hands below your shoulders and knees below your hips. Inhale to begin, then as you exhale, activate your deep core muscles as you raise one arm in front of you and extend the opposite leg. Hold for five to ten seconds, then switch sides. Do your best to keep your hips and shoulders aligned, rather than swaying to one side or the other.

The bird dog exercise may become uncomfortable later in pregnancy as your belly expands, but during the first half of pregnancy it's one of the best exercises for pain prevention. It not only activates the deepest layer of abdominal muscles but also strengthens the multifidus muscle, which plays a key role in stabilizing the spine.

Additional exercises that are considered safe during pregnancy and are very effective for core stabilization include glute bridges with your shoulders supported on an exercise ball or firm surface, and the Pallof press. To perform the latter, stand with a resistance band looped around a stable object to your side. The band should be at elbow height. Hold the end of the band with both hands close to your body. Take one or two steps to the side to create tension on the band, then activate your core as you exhale and push the band straight ahead of you, resisting the rotational pull of the band.

Exercises to Avoid

The main reason core exercises are treated with caution during pregnancy is concern about diastasis recti. This is a common condition involving separation of the abdominal muscles—specifically, the rectus abdominis, or six-pack muscles, which are held together by a band of connective tissue that runs down the center of the abdomen. During pregnancy, this area softens and stretches to accommodate a growing belly, usually creating a separation between the ab muscles that is around one finger's width. If the connective tissue becomes overstretched and weak, the separation may be much greater, and a wider gap may appear by the end of pregnancy. This condition, known as diastasis recti, can cause abdominal or back pain that may not resolve on its own after delivery.

Although women are often told to avoid all abdominal or core exercises while pregnant in order to avoid ab separation, only certain exercises pose a problem. Studies have found that women who perform exercises designed to strengthen the deep core abdominals tend to have a much lower chance of developing separation.[6] In one study run by physical therapists at Columbia University and Cedars-Sinai Medical Center, 90% of non-exercising women developed significant abdominal separation, compared to just 12.5% in those following an exercise program focused on strengthening the deep core abdominals.[7]

The best way to tell if a core exercise is problematic is by watching for a protrusion along the center line of the abdominals. If a pronounced bulge or ridge appears during a certain exercise, your abdominal muscles are likely under too much pressure and the exercise should be avoided or modified.

Which movements trigger this issue can vary from person to person, but experts typically recommend that pregnant women avoid crunches, sit-ups, twisting through the abdomen, and excessive backward arching. Additionally, it's best to roll to the side before sitting up in bed.

The long-standing advice to avoid crunches has been called into question more recently, with some studies showing that it activates muscles that may help address abdominal separation. However, this is likely only true if you're able to effectively turn on your deeper abdominal muscles.

Planks are another controversial exercise. Some physical therapists recommend avoiding standard front planks once your belly gets to a significant size unless you already have very good core strength. Side planks, on the other hand, are generally considered safe and are one of the best ways to activate the obliques and other muscles that stabilize your spine. If you do add side planks to your routine, it's important to begin each repetition by activating your transverse ab muscle to provide control and stability through your lower abdomen.

One common question is whether it's safe to perform exercises while lying on your back during pregnancy, given the traditional advice to avoid sleeping on your back during the second and third trimesters. This guidance is based on concern that the weight of the uterus can compress major blood vessels, limiting blood flow to the placenta and causing dizziness, lightheadedness, or nausea. MRI studies have shown that the difference in blood flow to the placenta while lying on your back is relatively minor,[8] so staying in this position for a short time while exercising is probably not a major concern if you feel comfortable. If you do start to feel dizzy or uncomfortable, many positions can be modified by propping yourself up so you're on a slight incline.

Preparing the Pelvic Floor for Labor

The pelvic floor is a group of muscles that acts as a sling to support the pelvic organs. Pregnant women are often advised to perform Kegel exercises to activate and strengthen these muscles. The purpose is to improve core stability, assist with labor, and prevent complications caused by pelvic floor dysfunction after birth, such as incontinence and pelvic organ prolapse. However, physical therapists in this area have started to question this advice, noting that the pelvic floor muscles are already activated when performing core exercises correctly—that is, with transverse ab activation. An isolated, strong contraction of the pelvic floor muscles in the form of a Kegel exercise is not a movement that naturally occurs in the real world and is probably not a necessary exercise during pregnancy. Performing the core exercises mentioned earlier is likely more helpful.

Many women also have tight, chronically activated pelvic floor muscles, which can cause weakness and dysfunction. Learning how to activate the pelvic floor is only half the equation, and it may be even more important to learn how to relax and lengthen these muscles. Doing so takes on particular importance toward the end of pregnancy because efficient pushing should involve actively contracting the transverse ab while relaxing and lengthening the pelvic floor. The goal is to reduce tension in the pelvic floor to create space for the baby to pass through the birth canal.

It can be helpful to have at least one appointment with a pelvic floor physical therapist at some point during your pregnancy so they can assess your baseline function and teach you the exercises that are most useful for your specific situation. Starting at around 35 weeks, most PTs recommend breathing exercises to help you learn how to relax the pelvic floor, along with stretches to lengthen these muscles. Commonly recommended stretches include deep squats, butterfly stretches, child's pose, and the happy baby yoga pose.

Key Points

- A strong core can help prevent back pain, shorten labor, and speed your recovery after you give birth.
- Core exercises should focus on activating the deep abdominal muscles that stabilize the spine.
- Recommended exercises include:
- transverse ab activation
- bird dog
- glute bridge with shoulders elevated
- Pallof press
- side plank
- To minimize ab separation, avoid exercises that cause a pronounced bulge along the midline of your abdomen.
- A functional pelvic floor is important, but Kegels may be unnecessary if you're performing core exercises correctly.
- Toward the end of the third trimester, learning to relax and lengthen your pelvic floor can help ensure an easier delivery.

PART 4

Evidence-Based Medical Care

Chapter 15

Pregnancy Vaccine Decisions

W E'RE LIVING IN an extraordinary time for vaccine breakthroughs. Until very recently, it was only possible to protect babies from whooping cough and flu. This is nothing to take for granted, and these vaccines no doubt save thousands of lives every year, but newborns were left vulnerable to another very common infection: respiratory syncytial virus (RSV). Now, thanks to decades of work by a team of determined researchers at the National Institutes of Health, we can finally protect babies from this illness.

This protection is important because newborns have very little ability to make their own antibodies until they are two to three months old. Contrary to popular myth, antibodies from breast milk don't offer much protection against respiratory infections, as discussed in more detail in Chapter 18. Your newborn's ability to fight infection is therefore heavily dependent on the antibodies transferred through the placenta during the later stages of pregnancy. This in turn depends on your own production of antibodies.

Although your immune system maintains a catalog of antibodies that recognize the thousands of microbes you've encountered, these antibodies are normally present in only tiny amounts. They serve as an early detection system, ready to alert the immune system in the event that a particular microbe is detected again, but they aren't present in sufficient numbers to neutralize an invading virus.

You're much more likely to transfer enough antibodies to protect your baby from an illness if you're actively making those antibodies—typically in response to a recent infection or vaccination. Even if you've been vaccinated against a particular illness before, getting another shot during pregnancy ramps up the production of antibodies so you can give your baby immune protection that will last for months after they're born.

If you aren't planning to get vaccinated during pregnancy, the best approach is to keep your baby home as much as possible in the early months, while their immune system is still developing. As you'll learn later in this chapter, it's also possible to protect against RSV with a new antibody treatment given directly to babies after they're born. Finally, we'll cover other ways to help ward off viruses and support your immune system so you can enjoy more of your pregnancy instead of succumbing to every cold and flu that passes by.

The RSV Vaccine Breakthrough

RSV is one of the most widespread and problematic viruses for infants. Half of all babies are infected by the time they turn one, and almost every child is infected at least once by age two. In adults, the virus typically causes mild symptoms similar to a cold or flu. In babies, particularly those under three months, RSV can be much more serious, often causing chest congestion that requires hospitalization. Before the advent of the new vaccine, RSV was the number one cause of hospitalization among infants. In North America and Europe, at least one in 50 healthy, full-term babies were hospitalized with RSV in their first year.[1]

This virus is so widespread because previous infection provides very little protection against future infections. If you catch RSV, you'll likely get just as sick the next time you're exposed. As a result, adults get RSV repeatedly throughout their lifetime, and there is never a shortage of people to pass along the virus.

The urgent need for a vaccine to protect babies from RSV was recognized soon after the virus was first identified in the 1950s, but this endeavor encountered one obstacle after another. Dozens of different RSV vaccines were developed and tested from the 1960s to the early 2000s, but all were abject failures.

Dr. Barney Graham at the NIH dedicated his life to solving this seemingly intractable problem, starting work on RSV vaccines in 1985. After more than 25 years of research, his big breakthrough came in 2013.

Dr. Graham, along with Dr. Jason McLellan and others at the NIH, finally figured out the shape that a critical protein on the surface of RSV takes right before the virus invades human cells. This discovery allowed them to use the protein in a vaccine to elicit the right kind of antibodies.

Known as the F protein, this molecule on the surface of the virus is "like a Transformer toy," Dr. Graham says. It's folded into one shape before the virus latches on to and invades a cell, and then unfolds and takes on another shape after the virus multiplies and breaks out. The first shape is known as the "prefusion" state, while the second is known as the "postfusion" state.

Drs. Graham and McLellan came up with the idea that a vaccine might be more successful if it was based on the prefusion shape. Antibodies could then recognize and neutralize the virus before it invaded. Because this form is extremely unstable and the protein spontaneously flips to the postfusion state when the virus is killed or inactivated, all prior vaccine attempts involved the postfusion form. After decades of failures, it was clear that vaccines based on this form of the protein simply didn't work.

In 2013, Drs. Graham and McLellan became the first to figure out the shape of the prefusion protein and how to modify it so it would remain locked in that form. With those discoveries, it suddenly became possible to develop a vaccine that could train the immune system to recognize the correct form of the F protein and block RSV from invading cells. This was an entirely new way of creating vaccines.

Drs. Graham and McLellan knew they'd finally found the answer when the first animal studies using their altered F protein showed an immune response vastly better than any prior RSV vaccines. The resulting antibodies had 50 times more neutralizing power against RSV than anything tested before. The critical decision was also made to vaccinate pregnant women rather than newborns. Instead of relying on a baby's own undeveloped immune system, antibodies from the mother could be passed along in utero, providing protection for several months after birth.

RSV Vaccine Timing

RSV rarely causes issues for healthy adults, even during pregnancy. That makes the timing relatively simple because the vaccine has only one main objective: producing antibodies to protect the baby after birth. To accomplish that goal, the best time to get the vaccine is toward the end of pregnancy, between 32 and 36 weeks.

Some countries allow for earlier vaccination, but this could be associated with a small increase in the chance of preterm birth.[2] In the initial clinical studies raising this concern, the increase wasn't statistically significant, and most premature births occurred around 36 weeks. Nevertheless, waiting until later in pregnancy has little downside, so the FDA and most experts recommend delaying until at least 32 weeks. The vaccine is given before the end of 36 weeks because it takes around two weeks for antibodies to be produced and transferred to the baby.

The official guidance in the United States also suggests limiting the RSV vaccine by season in most states. According to this approach, the vaccine is given to those who are 32–36 weeks pregnant between September and January in order to protect newborns during the peak RSV season.[3] In either very cold or tropical climates, RSV doesn't show the same seasonal patterns and can circulate at low levels throughout the year. In these areas, it likely makes sense to get vaccinated between 32 and 36 weeks regardless of the season.

If you won't be vaccinated during pregnancy because your expected delivery date is before or after RSV season, or if your baby arrives less than two weeks after you're vaccinated, there is fortunately another option to protect against the virus.

In years past, babies who were born prematurely and therefore at high risk for RSV infection were given an expensive antibody injection called Synagis. This treatment doesn't activate the baby's own immune system as a vaccine does, but instead provides antibodies made in the laboratory.

After injection with these antibodies, a baby is protected from serious illness in much the same way as if they had received maternal antibodies through the placenta. These lab-made antibodies don't last very long, though, so babies needed monthly injections. Given the high cost and logistical challenge, Synagis was reserved for only the highest-risk infants. In 2023, both problems were solved with the approval of a new single-dose antibody treatment that lasts the entire RSV season.

This one-time injection, called Beyfortus, is now recommended for all babies under eight months who were born during or are entering their first RSV season, if their mother didn't get the RSV vaccine at least two weeks before birth. [4]

Depending on the season, you may be given the choice of either getting vaccinated during pregnancy or having your baby receive an antibody injection after they're born. This is a matter of personal preference. Both options are very safe and effective, reducing the chance of severe RSV illness in the first three months by more than 80%.[5]

The Flu Vaccine

Another vaccine to consider during pregnancy is a flu shot. The flu is often considered a relatively mild and routine illness for healthy adults, but it can be worse during pregnancy. Changes to the immune system make it more difficult to clear the virus, so pregnant women often get sicker for longer. Additionally, there can be an exaggerated inflammatory response in the lungs, which can lead to hospitalization. The net effect is that pregnancy is associated with a seven-fold increase in the risk of being hospitalized with flu.[6] Getting vaccinated cuts this risk in half.[7] It also significantly lowers the risk of preterm birth.[8]

Because the flu vaccine has been given during pregnancy since the 1950s, we also have clear long-term data showing that it's safe and doesn't increase the risk of miscarriage or any other pregnancy complications.[9] One study suggested that vaccination in the first trimester could possibly be associated with a slightly higher rate of autism in children,[10] but the increase was not statistically significant, and subsequent studies have found no link.[11]

The official guidance from the CDC and American College of Obstetricians and Gynecologists (ACOG) advises that pregnant people should get vaccinated early in the flu season, regardless of their pregnancy stage. The national vaccination programs in some countries, such as Denmark and Norway, recommend waiting until the second or third trimester. This is not driven by a concern about safety or side effects, but rather maximizing protection for babies after they're born.

As with RSV, getting vaccinated against flu during pregnancy triggers the production of antibodies that will be transferred to your baby and protect against serious illness during the vulnerable newborn stage.[12] This transfer of antibodies through the placenta only begins at around 13 weeks. In the case of flu, the antibodies produced after vaccination also drop relatively quickly, so getting vaccinated later in the second trimester or in the third trimester gives babies much better protection.[13] This significantly reduces the chance of your newborn being hospitalized with flu.

In one study spanning more than 250,000 pregnancies, vaccination during pregnancy resulted in an 80% reduction in the chance of flu-related hospitalization in babies under six months.[14] In years when the vaccine is not as well matched to circulating strains, vaccination reduces the risk of infant hospitalization by about half.[15]

Even though waiting until the second or third trimester maximizes the transfer of antibodies to your baby, if your first trimester overlaps with peak flu season, it may still make sense to get vaccinated earlier to protect yourself from getting sick. This is a matter of weighing the pros and cons, depending on your health and the severity of the flu season.

Some people choose to get the flu and COVID vaccines together since the timing considerations are similar and the peak seasons for the two viruses tend to overlap.

Although not all vaccines can be combined, studies have found that getting these two shots on the same day doesn't significantly increase the risks and doesn't compromise the immune response to either vaccine.[16] The immune system is a master multitasker.

Another common question is whether a COVID booster is worthwhile for those who have already been vaccinated before pregnancy or who have natural immunity from a recent infection. This is a personal decision and a topic to discuss with your doctor, but the main advantage of getting vaccinated during pregnancy is a significant increase in the transfer of antibodies to your baby. This will help protect against serious infection in the first few months after they are born.[17]

The Tdap Vaccine During Pregnancy

The final vaccine routinely recommended during pregnancy is Tdap, which covers tetanus, diphtheria, and pertussis. The main reason to get this vaccine is the pertussis component, which aims to protect babies against whooping cough after they're born. Whooping cough is a highly contagious bacterial infection that can be life-threatening for infants. About one-third of babies who contract whooping cough end up in the hospital.

Vaccination during pregnancy is more than 90% effective, providing immunity to infants until they are at least two months old.[18] At that point, babies typically receive their own pertussis vaccine in the form of DTaP or another combination vaccine.

The standard advice is to get the Tdap vaccine when you are between 27 and 36 weeks pregnant, in every pregnancy. Studies have found, however, that we can likely optimize the transfer of antibodies to the baby by getting vaccinated during the earlier half of this window, between 28 and 32 weeks.[19]

Although the CDC and FDA advise that it's safe to receive multiple vaccines on the same day, even during pregnancy, it's likely best to get the Tdap vaccine on its own. Researchers have found that receiving the RSV vaccine at the same time as Tdap seems to reduce the effectiveness of the pertussis vaccine.[20] This provides another reason to get the Tdap vaccine earlier, at 28–32 weeks, and the RSV vaccine later, at around 34–35 weeks.

Other Ways to Support Your Immune System

Although vaccines are one of the most powerful tools we have to protect against infections, they can't prevent every illness. Fortunately, there are other ways to support your immune system and reduce the chance of getting sick.

One of the most effective strategies is ensuring that you have adequate vitamin D levels throughout pregnancy. Vitamin D not only boosts your ability to fight infections so you're less likely to get sick, but also helps prevent complications by calming the part of the immune system responsible for inflammation. It is this inflammation that typically links severe illness and pregnancy complications. Studies have found that pregnant women with vitamin D deficiency are over five times more likely to develop severe COVID.[21] By contrast, those with sufficient vitamin D levels tend to have much milder symptoms and are less likely to develop downstream complications such as preeclampsia.[22]

Another simple but effective strategy to lower the chance of getting sick and speed up recovery time is to use a saline nasal spray. These aerosol sprays, consisting of pure salt water, can be found in supermarkets and pharmacies under brand names such as Simply Saline.

Researchers have found that using a saline nasal spray signif-icantly reduces viral load and allows you to clear viruses more quickly. One study reported that when people with COVID starting using a nasal spray soon after they tested positive, more than 90% had cleared the virus within ten days, compared to just 28% in matched controls.[23] This strategy is most effective if the spray is used approximately every three hours, but just once or twice per day also makes a difference.[24] By helping to clear the virus quickly, nasal irrigation also appears to reduce the risk of hospitalization. One study of high-risk patients who tested positive for COVID found that those using saline nasal spray were eight times less likely to be hospitalized.[25]

For even greater effect, you can gargle with warm salt water for 60 seconds several times per day. This reduces the viral load in the throat by nearly 90%.[26]

These strategies can also be used preventively. Studies of health care workers and those exposed to COVID from household members suggest that daily saline spray can significantly reduce the chance of getting sick.[27] The same is likely true for the flu, the common cold, and other viruses.[28] If you seem to catch every illness that goes around, you might consider adding a quick saline nasal rinse to your bedtime routine to increase the odds of staying healthy, especially in winter.

If you still end up getting sick and find yourself very congested, the medication options during pregnancy can be rather limited, particularly if you have high blood pressure. One of the best solutions is to use a saline spray with a higher salt content to help you quickly clear the congestion and breathe more easily.

Key Points

- Getting the RSV vaccine when you're between 32 and 36 weeks will help protect your newborn from this very common virus. It is typically offered to those who will deliver during or shortly before RSV season. Alternatively, your baby can receive their own antibody shot.

- Getting vaccinated against flu and COVID during pregnancy will transfer antibodies to your baby to protect them from serious illness during the vulnerable newborn stage.

- The optimal timing for these vaccines depends on how your pregnancy overlaps with the peak viral season, but they provide more protection to your baby if you're vaccinated in the second or third trimester.

- Getting the Tdap vaccine during pregnancy aims to protect babies against whooping cough after they're born. The optimal time for this vaccine is 28—32 weeks.

- Maintaining good vitamin D levels and using a saline nasal spray can reduce the odds of getting sick and help you recover sooner.

Chapter 16

Third-Trimester Monitoring and Induction

W HEN YOU REACH the later stages of the third trimester, the level of monitoring you'll receive can
vary depending on your risk factors, your doctor's
approach to screening, and even which country you live in. If
you live in the U.S. and conceived at a later age, or with relevant medical history, you'll typically have frequent monitoring
in the final months of pregnancy. This may involve ultrasound
measurements, assessing amniotic fluid levels, and tracking
the baby's heart rate during so-called non-stress tests. All
these screening methods offer indirect ways of assessing fetal
growth, fetal well-being, and whether the placenta is keeping
up with the baby's needs.

In low-risk pregnancies, and in countries with a more
hands-off approach to obstetrics, these tests may not be
offered unless an issue is flagged. Instead, you'll typically be
advised to monitor your baby's movements by way of kick

counting. You can do this in various ways. One is to choose a time each day when the baby is active. Lie down on your left side and note how long it takes for you to feel 10 movements. You can record this information in an app, such as Count the Kicks. It's best to start counting kicks from the beginning of the third trimester so you can learn your baby's patterns and become more aware of anything out of the ordinary.

Kick counting sounds like a low-tech, old-fashioned way to monitor your baby's health, but it works. Studies have demonstrated that it can be one of the best ways to identify problems early enough for a baby in distress to be delivered safely.[1] When a campaign to encourage kick counting was introduced in Iowa, the state's stillbirth rate dropped by a third, while the rates remained steady in the rest of the country.[2] Your doctor is likely aware of this data and the importance of monitoring fetal movement, so if you notice a change, you shouldn't worry about coming across as overly anxious or bothering anyone with false alarms. It's always better to err on the side of checking to make sure everything is fine.

Even if all is going well as you approach your due date and no concerns are raised by third trimester monitoring or decreased movement, your doctor may recommend an induction at 39 or 40 weeks as a precaution, particularly if you're over 35 or conceived by IVF. This recommendation often comes as a surprise and may seem like an unnecessary intervention, but it's something to genuinely consider.

The tide is shifting more in favor of induction following recent studies that found a significantly lower rate of stillbirths and other complications when labor is induced at or after 39 weeks, even in the lowest-risk pregnancies.[3] The benefits of induction are likely even greater for those with risk factors related to the placenta, such as advanced maternal age, low amniotic fluid, or fetal growth restriction.[4]

The most recent studies are also alleviating some of the concerns over induction, such as whether starting down this path may increase the odds of needing a C-section. As this chapter explains, a body of research has now shown that induction may in fact reduce the odds of needing a C-section. That is likely because delivering earlier can avoid many of the complications that can disrupt plans for a vaginal delivery. For mothers with gestational diabetes, for example, induction can reduce the chance of needing a C-section due to the baby's size.

Nevertheless, the risks and benefits are not always clear-cut, and factors such as an uncertain due date or a desire for an unmedicated birth can come into play. In the end, whether to have an induction is a decision to make with your doctor, taking into account your unique circumstances and preferences. To make a truly informed decision, third-trimester monitoring can be valuable, providing insight into how well your baby is growing and how well your placenta is functioning.

Measuring Baby's Growth

In years past, a common method of tracking a baby's growth was to measure the mother's belly from the pubic bone to the top of the uterus, called the fundus. As you might expect, this simplistic method is not a reliable way to identify problems with the placenta or a baby's growth.[5] Ultrasound measurement is slightly better but still prone to error because the machines become less accurate as babies get bigger. Many parents are told their baby is measuring either very big or very small, only to have a perfectly average-size baby arrive a few weeks later. The most reliable ultrasound measurement appears to be the baby's abdominal circumference, but even this has limited ability to predict whether a baby is large for gestational age or has fetal growth restriction, and false alarms are common.[6] For that reason, doctors typically look at the whole picture, including changes in growth pattern over time and other factors such as the amount of amniotic fluid and the baby's activity level.

Measuring Amniotic Fluid

The main reason to assess the level of amniotic fluid is to determine whether the placenta is functioning well and supporting the baby's growth. Amniotic fluid provides an insight into the functioning of the placenta because it's made by your baby's kidneys. Normal amniotic fluid levels are a good sign that your placenta is healthy and your baby is receiving all the blood flow and nutrients needed.

The amount of amniotic fluid is typically estimated at each ultrasound in the third trimester. If the fluid seems low, your doctor will try to get a fuller picture by checking your baby's heart rate and activity level. If these other tests suggest an issue, an earlier induction will likely be recommended out of an abundance of caution.

If fluid is low but your baby's growth and activity are normal, there is little evidence that an induction is necessary, but doctors typically err on the side of recommending induction if you're close to full term. At that point, there's no reason to take the chance of waiting, and the safest option is to deliver sooner.

Sometimes amniotic fluid may be low simply because you're dehydrated. This can reduce blood flow to the placenta, reducing the output of amniotic fluid from the baby's kidneys.[7] To avoid this situation, make sure you're staying well hydrated during the third trimester, especially before ultrasound appointments.

Studies show that consuming two liters of water in the hours before an ultrasound can avoid many cases of low amniotic fluid measurements. An even better strategy is to drink at least two liters of water as a daily habit.[8] When this is done for at least a week before an ultrasound, many women who otherwise would have been diagnosed with low amniotic fluid are found to have normal fluid levels.[9]

Non-Stress Tests

In a non-stress test, a fetal heart monitor band is placed around your belly and used to measure the baby's heart rate for around 20 minutes to half an hour. This test looks for variations in heart rate that indicate the baby is moving and active. When the baby moves, their heart rate briefly accelerates. If accelerations aren't present, the test is considered "nonreactive," meaning the heart rate is remaining steady because the baby isn't moving around much.

Most often, this is simply because the baby is sleeping. Your doctor will usually wait for the baby to wake up before repeating the test. To encourage your little one to stay awake, you can try making a loud noise, such as by clapping close to the belly, or eating dark chocolate.[10] Researchers have also found that music helps keep many babies awake and active enough to pass their non-stress tests.[11]

If you fall into any of the higher-risk categories, your doctor may recommend a weekly non-stress test or ultrasound, or both, starting at around 32 weeks. Although this can be time-consuming and inconvenient, the approach is supported by both the scientific research and the official guidelines from Maternal Fetal Medicine specialists.[12] Weekly monitoring can help identify problems early so the baby can be delivered if needed and so you can be reassured that all is going well.

Measuring the Placenta

Another potential tool for assessing whether the placenta is providing sufficient nourishment, or whether a baby may need to be delivered sooner, is to measure the placenta directly. At the time of writing, few doctors are offering this screening, even though it simply involves taking a few measurements of the placenta during a standard ultrasound and entering those measurements into an online calculator to estimate the total volume.[13]

Harvey J. Kliman, M.D., Ph.D., the director of the Reproductive and Placental Research Unit at Yale, would like to change that and see placenta measurement become more routine so problems can be identified sooner and more babies can be delivered safely.

In Dr. Kliman's research, the single most common cause of unexplained stillbirth is a very small placenta.[14] It's logical to expect that identifying these cases in time could make a difference, but we don't yet have definitive proof of that from clinical trials. Given how rare stillbirth is, any such trial would need to be very large and involve a huge investment of resources. In the absence of such a trial, organizations such as ACOG are reluctant to recommend measuring the placenta, and few obstetricians are willing to depart from the official guidelines.

Nevertheless, if signs indicate that your placenta may not be functioning well, if you have experienced unexplained late-term pregnancy loss or intrauterine growth restriction, or if you have a medical condition such as diabetes or a blood clotting disorder, it may be worth discussing this potential screening method with your obstetrician or a maternal fetal medicine or high-risk pregnancy specialist. Measure the Placenta, an organization dedicated to raising awareness of this issue, also provides resources for physicians and patients and a list of providers on their website at measuretheplacenta.org.

Routine Induction

Even if all signs are positive and no issues are flagged during any of the third-trimester monitoring, your doctor may still recommend induction once you reach 39 or 40 weeks rather than waiting for you to go into labor naturally.

In the United States, inductions are performed in more than a quarter of deliveries. That percentage has been growing in recent years as more research has emerged that shows induction can reduce the odds of stillbirth. By delivering at 39 or 40 weeks, it's possible to avoid the pregnancy losses that would occur after that point, whether due to infections, cord accidents, or deterioration of the placenta.[15] Delivering earlier makes the most difference if you have any risk factors related to the placenta, but even in the lowest-risk pregnancies, a significant body of data favors induction once you reach 39 weeks.[16]

The threshold is usually set at 39 weeks for low-risk pregnancies because at 37 and 38 weeks, the lungs are still in the final stages of maturing, and babies born around this time may need more help with breathing or maintaining their blood sugar levels.[17] After 39 weeks, however, a baby is considered full term, and staying pregnant longer doesn't significantly improve infant health outcomes.[18]

Previously, it was thought that remaining in utero until 40 or 41 weeks improved a baby's brain development, but the most recent studies suggest otherwise. Induction at 39 weeks appears to have no negative impact on cognitive development or any other measures of brain function later in childhood.[19]

The challenge with setting the threshold at 39 weeks and inducing at any time after that point is that not all pregnancies can be dated accurately. If your doctor is unsure of your exact due date, that weighs in favor of waiting a little longer to ensure that your baby is ready. On the other hand, if you conceived through IVF, your due date can be determined very accurately, and there is less reason to wait.

Another common concern is that labor may not progress well following an induction, increasing the chance of a C-section. This concern was eased significantly with the publication of the ARRIVE trial, which found that induction in low-risk pregnancies at 39 weeks was actually associated with a *lower* chance of needing a C-section.[20] Since then, numerous other studies have reported a similar pattern.[21] This is likely because the longer a pregnancy continues, the more opportunity exists to develop high blood pressure or another condition that may necessitate a C-section.[22]

A variety of methods can be used to induce labor, ranging from procedures and medications given in your doctor's office to a formal induction in the hospital. One of the procedures your doctor may offer in their office is a membrane sweep, which helps separate part of the amniotic sac from the wall of the uterus. This procedure promotes the release of hormones and prostaglandins that soften and dilate the cervix and stimulate contractions. Although the procedure can be painful and doesn't always make a difference, for many women it can trigger labor within two days.

In a formal induction, the process can vary depending on how close you are to going into labor on your own. This is reflected in the Bishop score, which is calculated from a combination of measures such as how much your cervix has dilated and thinned, and whether the baby's head has dropped down. If your Bishop score is over eight, indicating that you're ready for labor, the induction process may begin with an I.V. drip with Pitocin. This is a synthetic version of the hormone oxytocin, which works by stimulating contractions. If your Bishop score is lower, the first step may be a medication such as Cytotec or Cervidil. These medications mimic a natural signaling molecule known as prostaglandin E2, which helps dilate the cervix and prepare the body for labor. Pitocin may then be given as a second step to stimulate contractions. Doctors can also break your water to encourage labor to progress, but this is usually only done once active labor starts because if the baby isn't born within 24 hours, the chance of infection starts to rise.

Many other natural methods are purported to help kickstart labor, but the research indicates that most are not very effective.[23] The strategy most likely to have an impact is walking. One study found that when women nearing their due date walked for at least 30 minutes, three times per week, only 18% required an induction, compared to 33% of those not walking regularly.[24]

Key Points

- Monitoring during the third trimester aims to assess whether your placenta is meeting all the baby's needs and this helps guide decisions on whether induction may be warranted.

- Even if all is going well and your pregnancy is low risk, there could be some advantage to inducing at 39 or 40 weeks. This is a decision to make with your doctor, taking into account any uncertainty about your expected due date.

- Induction after 39 weeks is associated with a lower chance of needing a C-section than waiting until you go into labor naturally.

- Your doctor may be able to prompt labor without a formal induction by performing a membrane sweep.

- The natural method with the best chance of kick-starting labor is walking for at least 30 minutes three times a week.

Chapter 17

Delivery Decisions

C HILDBIRTH CAN BE unpredictable and does not always go according to plan, but you will have experts at your side ready to guide you through every step of the process. Whether you plan to deliver with an obstetrician, midwife, or a whole team of practitioners, there will be someone helping you navigate any challenges and decision points that may arise.

Even so, it's worth giving some thought to your preferences ahead of time. For in-depth guidance, it may be helpful to complete a childbirth course through your hospital or birth center, or with a midwife or doula, so you can find out what options and choices are available where you'll deliver. To complement that guidance, this chapter covers the pros and cons of epidurals, the rationale behind antibiotics during labor, the benefits of delayed cord clamping, and what to expect from a C-section.

In the end, your delivery may not go exactly as you expected, but it's just a tiny fraction of your experience as a parent. What matters most is protecting your health and ensuring your baby's safe arrival, however they end up coming into the world.

The Pros and Cons of Epidurals

Although many aspects of labor and delivery are hard to predict, one decision usually within your control is whether to get an epidural. Used in more than 70% of hospital deliveries, epidurals are generally regarded as the safest and most effective pain-relief option during childbirth. The procedure involves a quick numbing shot, after which the doctor places a tiny plastic tube into the lower spine. Numbing medication can then be delivered through the tube as needed during labor.

Epidurals pose little to no risk to the baby's health because the medication acts locally and does not cross the placenta. In contrast, some pain medications, such as opioids, can potentially slow a baby's breathing after birth.

For the mother, epidurals are also quite safe. The main risk is a severe headache, which occurs less than 1% of the time.[1] Low blood pressure and fever are slightly more common. In decades past, some concern existed that epidurals could slow labor and potentially increase the need for a C-section, vacuum assistance, or forceps delivery, but this has been refuted by more recent studies.[2] In one interesting natural experiment, researchers looked at the rate of C-sections in a Hawaii military hospital after a policy change resulted in a sudden increase in epidurals, soaring from 1% to more than 80% of deliveries in the span of a year. Over that time, there was no increase in the need for C-sections, vacuum assistance, or forceps.[3] Labor was slightly longer after epidurals were introduced—by approximately 25 minutes—but this doesn't have much practical impact.

The main disadvantage of having an epidural is that you'll have less ability to move around and be active during labor. With modern epidurals that use a lower dose of numbing medication, you typically have more feeling and can move your legs and change positions, but you'll be unsteady on your feet, so most hospitals have you stay in bed.

If you're still undecided on whether to get an epidural, you can typically make the decision after labor begins. Unless your labor progresses very rapidly, you'll have a substantial window of time in which to opt for one. With most doctors, this starts from when you are a couple of centimeters dilated until shortly before you're fully dilated and ready to push. "I have done epidurals at one centimeter and when a woman is fully dilated at 10 centimeters," says Dr. PJ McGuire, an obstetric anesthesiologist at Yale University.

The main limitations at later stages of labor are the availability of an anesthesiologist, your ability to hold still for the procedure, and the time it takes for the epidural to work. Placement of an epidural can take 10–15 minutes, and then another 15 minutes or more to work. If you're fully dilated and ready to push, an epidural may not be worthwhile because your baby will likely be born before it takes effect.

Even when it's too late for an epidural, other pain-relief options are usually available, including a spinal block, IV medications, or nitrous oxide gas. Not all hospitals offer nitrous oxide, and it's not effective for everyone, but some patients find it works well enough to substitute for an epidural.

Antibiotics During Labor

Antibiotics are given during labor approximately 40% of the time.[4] One reason is that many women have a higher body temperature during labor because epidurals compromise the ability to cool down by sweating. Antibiotics are typically given in this situation in case the higher body temperature is from an infection. Antibiotics are also routinely given during labor to prevent the transfer of group B strep to the baby.

About 25% of women carry this bacterium. Although it generally causes no symptoms in adults, in rare cases it can be dangerous for babies who acquire it during birth. As a result, the CDC recommends screening for group B strep at 35 to 37 weeks. For those who test positive, IV antibiotics are given during labor, ideally every four hours until the baby is born.

This treatment has the potential to impact your baby's microbiome by reducing the transfer of beneficial microbes during birth, but the need to protect babies from serious infection takes priority.[5] Overall, the downsides of receiving antibiotics during labor are minimal compared to the risks of a group B strep infection in a newborn.[6]

The good news is that specific probiotics may reduce the odds of testing positive for strep and therefore avoid the need for antibiotics. The probiotics that appear to have the most impact are *L. rhamnosus* GR-1 and *L. reuteri* RC-14. These strains have been the subject of research for more than 30 years. During that time, numerous studies have demonstrated that these probiotics help maintain a healthier vaginal flora.[7] The combination is offered by various brands, including

Jarrow Fem-Dophilus, RepHresh Pro-B, and OptiBac for Women Probiotics. Although many probiotics are adapted to the gastrointestinal tract, these strains are tailor-made to survive and persist in the female reproductive system. There they create a healthier pH and combat a variety of harmful microbes, including yeast and group B strep.

Studies have found that taking GR-1 and RC-14 during the third trimester may reduce the odds of testing positive for group B strep. In one of the larger studies on this subject, 40% of the women taking the probiotic tested negative for group B strep, compared to only 18% in the placebo group.[8] Other studies have found a smaller effect, or no effect at all, but these used a lower dose of one capsule per day instead of the recommended two.[9]

You can start this probiotic at any time during pregnancy, but for the purposes of preventing group B strep, it is likely only necessary during the third trimester. If you struggle with frequent yeast infections or other microbial imbalances, it may be preferable to start the probiotic earlier.

When to Cut the Cord

The conventional approach has always been to clamp and cut the umbilical cord within the first minute after birth. This was assumed to limit maternal blood loss and reduce the risk of hemorrhage, but there was never much evidence supporting this belief. In reality, the timing of cord clamping seems to make no real difference to the mother's health.[10]

The timing does, however, make a difference for the baby. Before birth, around 30% of the baby's blood is flowing through the placenta at any given time. If the cord is clamped immediately after birth, much of this blood is left behind in the placenta, reducing the baby's supply of iron-rich blood cells. A delay of several minutes allows more blood to be transferred, which helps in building up the baby's iron stores. This has a lasting positive impact, with higher iron levels still evident 12 months later.[11]

In addition to reducing the chance of anemia, a greater supply of iron during the first year plays a surprisingly important role in brain development.[12] Research has found that iron is needed to produce myelin, the fatty insulation that wraps around neurons and helps them transmit signals efficiently. When doctors wait several minutes before cord clamping, babies show improved myelination at four months old.[13] This likely translates into lasting cognitive benefits.

Thankfully, this is one area in which the official guidelines were quickly updated to reflect new research findings. In 2017, the American College of Obstetricians and Gynecologists (ACOG) issued an opinion recommending a delay in cord clamping for at least 30–60 seconds after birth. The opinion states that "delayed umbilical cord clamping increases hemoglobin levels at birth and improves iron stores in the first several months of life, which may have a favorable effect on developmental outcomes."[14] In premature babies, recent studies indicate that an even greater benefit is seen when clamping is delayed by at least two minutes.[15]

Although the practice of delayed cord clamping has now been widely adopted, not all obstetricians follow the guidelines. In recent surveys, about 80% of doctors routinely practice delayed cord clamping, although half delay only up to 30 seconds.[16] You can ask your doctor about their standard practice and let them know your preference.

For those who wish to do so, storing or donating your baby's cord blood should be possible even with delayed cord clamping. One of the main cord blood banks in the United States, Cord Blood Registry (CBR), reports that "in our experience, healthcare providers have been able to collect a sufficient volume of cord blood for storage even when practicing delayed cord clamping, giving your baby the best of both opportunities."[17]

C-Sections

It's natural to feel disappointed if your doctor recommends a C-section when you were hoping for a vaginal delivery, but it's often the safest path for you and your baby.

C-sections are performed in around one-third of deliveries, usually for medical reasons such as the size or position of the baby, problems with the progression of labor, or the position of the placenta. The procedure is even more likely to be necessary in women who are pregnant in their late 30s or early 40s, when conditions such as gestational diabetes, placenta previa, and preeclampsia become more common.[18]

One of the primary concerns about having a C-section is the potential for a longer postpartum recovery. You'll likely have some abdominal pain or tenderness for several days or weeks, but the recovery is often less difficult than many people expect. A C-section is much like a vaginal delivery in that some recoveries are quick and easy while others are more challenging. That said, most women who undergo a C-section can manage with over-the-counter pain relievers such as Tylenol or ibuprofen from the second or third day after delivery. Moving around and walking regularly can also speed the recovery process.

Another common reason for disappointment about needing a C-section is that it can seem like a more clinical and less natural way to welcome your baby into the world. But those moments matter far less than the thousands of other moments you and your baby will spend together. Planned C-sections can also be more relaxed and joyous than you might think. You'll normally be awake and only feel some tugging and pressure. Your partner will likely be with you, and a nurse may offer to play music and take photos. The whole procedure will be over quickly, and you'll usually be able to see and hold your baby soon after they are born.

Delivering by C-section can possibly lead to a longer delay before your milk comes in and may potentially impact your baby's microbiome, but the effects are relatively minor and there are ways to address any issues. If your milk is delayed, pumping regularly and having more skin-to-skin time with your baby can make a significant difference. Supplementing with formula for the first few days also has little downside, as the next chapter explains. It's also possible to support your baby's microbiome after a C-section, as you'll learn in Chapter 20.

Key Points

- Epidurals are considered the safest and most effective method for pain relief during labor.

- The probiotic strains *L. rhamnosus* GR-1 and *L. reuteri* RC-14 may reduce the odds of needing antibiotics during labor by reducing colonization with group B strep.

- Delayed cord clamping helps increase your baby's supply of iron-rich blood cells, which benefits long-term brain development.

- There is a one-in-three chance you'll need a C-section, but the procedure itself and the postpartum recovery phase will likely be easier than you expect.

PART 5

Caring for Your Newborn

Chapter 18

Breastfeeding and the Formula Wars

BREAST MILK IS no doubt one of the best sources of nutrition for babies, but formula also has its time and place. The highest priority, especially in the first few days, is making sure your baby receives enough nutrition, whatever the source.

Sometimes efforts to encourage breastfeeding can create unnecessary fear around giving formula, but the most recent studies show that it's possible to supplement with formula without compromising your chance of successful breastfeeding. It's also becoming evident that the benefits of breastfeeding are less significant than initially thought and that the impact of dehydration and low blood sugar in newborns deserves more attention.

The Evidence on Breastfeeding

The purported benefits of breastfeeding include lower rates of asthma, eczema, allergy, obesity, and infections, along with higher IQ scores. But when we look at all the evidence, these benefits appear somewhat exaggerated, causing unnecessary guilt for parents who are unable to breastfeed or find they need to supplement with formula.

One of the most high-profile studies on the subject is the PROBIT trial, which tracked breastfeeding among 14,000 mother-infant pairs. The study found that breastfeeding did not reduce the risk of respiratory infections, asthma, allergies, or attention-deficit hyperactivity disorder (ADHD).[1] It did, however, slightly reduce gastrointestinal infections and improve cognitive development.

These two specific benefits—to the GI system and the brain—are the most consistent findings among the many other studies evaluating breastfeeding versus formula feeding. In another example, researchers compared various health outcomes and vocabulary scores among 500 sibling pairs where only one sibling was breastfed.[2] On respiratory infections, asthma, and allergies, the researchers found that breastfeeding made little difference. For the most part, "the long-term effects of breast feeding have been overstated," the authors wrote.

Yet the children who were breastfed scored higher on vocabulary tests, indicating that breast milk provides additional benefits for cognitive development. This finding is consistent with more than a dozen other studies finding higher cognitive scores in breastfed infants, with even greater benefits with longer duration of breastfeeding.[3]

Through the sea of conflicting information in this area, there is one other relatively consistent finding: a slight reduction in gastrointestinal infections.[4] When it comes to other types of infections, the benefits of breastfeeding are often exaggerated on the basis of a common misconception about how the human immune system works.

Many people believe that breastfeeding offers powerful immune benefits because antibodies are transferred through colostrum and milk from mother to baby. That's not actually true, as explained by Dr. Sydney Spiesel, a pediatrician and clinical professor at Yale University's School of Medicine:

When you ask a bunch of doctors about how breastfeeding prevents infection, they get it wrong—I know they do, because I've asked the question. Doctors tell you that colostrum (produced in the first three days or so after a baby is born) and breast milk are full of maternal antibodies. Next, doctors say that these maternal antibodies are absorbed into the infant's blood circulation and thus serve to protect infants from disease.[5]

That's true for most mammals, but not humans. Breast milk is rich in antibodies, but babies can't absorb these antibodies into the bloodstream in any significant amount.[6] As Dr. Spiesel notes:

Human babies are never able to absorb maternal antibodies from milk or colostrum into the bloodstream, except perhaps in the minutest amounts. Maternal antibodies in milk and colostrum protect against infection—but only locally, working inside the baby's gastrointestinal tract.

In other words, the antibodies from breast milk generally remain in your baby's digestive system. There they may help prevent some infections, but this is far from the protective force field many people imagine.

Yet that doesn't mean a newborn is left defenseless. Unlike other animals, humans are already born with the powerful protection of their mother's antibodies. During the third trimester, these antibodies are transferred across the placenta into the infant's bloodstream.[7] They remain there and provide protection from birth until the baby's own immune system develops during the first few months of life. "That's why we don't need to absorb maternal antibodies from colostrum. And it's why formula-fed babies are not at a disadvantage, compared with breast-fed babies, in their supply of circulating maternal antibodies," Spiesel notes.[8]

Early studies finding reduced rates of ear infections and upper respiratory infections in breastfed infants were likely plagued by a problem known as "confounding." This means that some additional factor other than breastfeeding was the true cause of lower infection rates in breastfed infants.

This pattern was shown in a recent study that categorized mothers by whether or not they *intended* to breastfeed. The mothers who had every intention of nursing had children with fewer infections, even if they didn't actually end up breastfeeding. The study authors commented that "the same characteristics that lead a mother to breastfeed may also lead to an infant having improved health."[9] As explained by Dr. Amy Tuteur, obstetrician and author of *Push Back: Guilt in the Age of Natural Parenting*, "It is the differences between mothers that are responsible for the differences in outcome, not breastfeeding."[10]

Another often-cited benefit of breastfeeding is a lower rate of asthma, eczema, and allergies. The evidence on this point is somewhat inconsistent. One review noted that less than half the studies on this subject found a benefit from breastfeeding, whereas the rest reported no difference.[11] A more recent systematic review concluded that "there is some evidence that breastfeeding is protective for asthma . . . There is weaker evidence for a protective effect for eczema."[12]

If breastfeeding does indeed help prevent these conditions, it's likely by way of supporting the microbiome, the population of beneficial microbes in the gastrointestinal tract. We know that breast milk helps "seed" a baby's microbiome with beneficial bacteria such as lactobacilli and bifidobacteria—microbes that play a critical role in educating the immune system.

We also know that breast milk contains a wide variety of indigestible carbohydrates, also known as *pre*biotics, which are present solely to nurture gut microbes. The net result is that babies who are breastfed typically have a more robust population of beneficial microbes and fewer harmful ones.[13] This in turn may reduce the rates of allergy and eczema in breastfed babies because these microbes serve to train the immune system.[14]

Yet the major studies in this area were performed before formula manufacturers began adding prebiotics in an effort to mimic the beneficial effects of breast milk on the microbiome. As discussed in more detail in Chapter 19, by choosing a formula containing prebiotics and supplementing with the right probiotics, we can build a microbiome very similar to that of a breastfed infant, resulting in similar rates of food allergy, eczema, and other immune conditions.[15]

Supporting the microbiome in this way also appears to reduce the number of gastrointestinal infections, mimicking another potential advantage of breastfeeding. By building a healthier population of beneficial species using probiotics and prebiotics, the harmful species that cause gastrointestinal infections have less opportunity to take hold.

Breastfeeding still has an apparent advantage over formula when it comes to supporting a baby's growing brain, but here, too, recent developments in formula development are starting to close the gap.

Effects on Brain Development

Initially, it was thought that breast milk was uniquely beneficial for brain development due to its higher proportion of omega-3 fatty acids, particularly DHA. For this reason, manufacturers have been adding DHA to infant formula for many years. However, the benefits in terms of cognitive development have been somewhat disappointing.

As discussed in Chapter 2, a steady supply of DHA during pregnancy is crucial for brain development. Breastfed infants also typically show higher levels of DHA than formula-fed infants as long as the mother has adequate intake.[16] But the addition of DHA to formula doesn't seem to lessen the gap between formula and breast milk when it comes to supporting brain development.[17]

More recently, formula manufacturers have developed a new way to replicate some of the brain-boosting effects of breast milk by adding a component known as milk fat globule membrane (MFGM). This is a combination of lipids and proteins that forms a membrane around fat droplets in breast milk. MFGM is also present in cow's milk, but it used to be discarded along with the milk fat when manufacturing infant formula. That changed when researchers discovered that MFGM contains several components that could be helpful for brain development.[18] As a result, MFGM is now included in several brands of infant formula, as discussed in more detail in the next chapter.

Taking a step back, it's likely that breast milk is still the best choice for nourishing babies. But formula is getting closer than ever, and the benefits of breastfeeding are less significant than suggested by many experts. This is important to recognize because many mothers are unable to breastfeed for as long as they would like—or at all—or they may need to supplement with formula.

The World Health Organization recommends exclusive breastfeeding for six months, but in the United States, only a quarter of mothers manage that feat.[19] Most women stop breastfeeding earlier than they would like, due to factors such as illnesses requiring medication, unsupportive work policies, and lack of parental leave.

If you are one of the 75% of parents who need to feed your baby formula at some point, take comfort in the knowledge that you're still providing a perfectly good source of nutrition.

Early Formula Supplementation and the Fed Is Best Campaign

Supplementing with formula takes on even greater importance when there is a significant delay in milk supply. These delays are surprisingly common: up to 15% of first-time mothers don't produce enough milk to meet their baby's needs, particularly in the first few days after birth.[20] Risk factors include Cesarean delivery, severe bleeding after birth, diabetes, PCOS, obesity, thyroid conditions, and prolonged bed rest during pregnancy.[21]

Unfortunately, the problem of delayed milk supply is not taken seriously enough, out of fear of interfering with the delicate process of nursing. Many hospitals and health professionals are eager to encourage breastfeeding at all costs. This sometimes leads them to discourage supplementing with formula even when infants truly need it.

This single-minded focus on breastfeeding can put babies at risk. If milk production is significantly delayed, a newborn can quickly become dehydrated and experience low blood glucose levels. In extreme cases, this can have a long-term impact on a baby's brain. Severe low blood sugar in newborns, known as neonatal hypoglycemia, is in fact the most common preventable cause of brain damage in infancy.

One of the leading crusaders in this area is Dr. Christie del Castillo-Hegyi. In addition to being an emergency-room physician, former NIH scientist, and newborn brain injury researcher, she is also the mother of a child who became neurologically disabled due to insufficient milk intake in the first days of life.[22] Her heartbreaking story is unfortunately not unique. Numerous other cases have been reported where exclusively breastfed babies developed severe low blood glucose levels between the second and fifth day of life from insufficient milk intake.[23]

Dr. del Castillo-Hegyi now works to spread this message to parents, hospitals, pediatricians, and government policymakers through the nonprofit she founded: the Fed Is Best Foundation. Her most important message: "Safely meeting an infant's full nutritional need is more important than exclusively breastfeeding."

In some cases, determining whether a newborn requires supplementation can be a finely balanced decision. But the studies do not support the common view, urged by some lactation consultants, that supplementing with formula harms the chance of success with breastfeeding. In fact, the opposite may be true.

A randomized study led by Dr. Valerie Flaherman at the University of California, San Francisco, found that supplementing with formula after each breastfeeding session from the first day after birth until the mother's milk supply is fully established had no negative impact on the likelihood of successful breastfeeding at three months.[24] Doing so also had clear benefits, reducing both the risk of dehydration and low blood sugar and the odds of a newborn being readmitted to the hospital for conditions such as jaundice.[25]

In addition, supplementing with formula when breast milk is inadequate can have more subtle benefits for brain development.[26] Even when blood sugar isn't low enough to cause significant neurological impairment, there can be a negative impact on cognitive function.

Researchers have found that a baby who has very low blood glucose levels within the first 24 hours is five times more likely to have lower motor, cognitive, and language scores at one year of age. [27] These negative effects are still apparent many years later. At age four, these young children are more likely to face problems with planning, memory, attention, problem-solving, and motor function.[28]

Although the vast majority of exclusively breastfed infants receive adequate nutrition and don't need formula supplementation, it's helpful to be fully informed about what to watch for so you can act quickly at the first signs of a problem with early milk supply.

This is particularly important if you have one of the risk factors for insufficient milk supply, namely:[29]

- delivery by C-section
- hypothyroidism
- polycystic ovarian syndrome
- minimal growth of breast tissue during pregnancy
- history of infertility
- advanced maternal age
- autoimmune disease
- retained placenta

The main warning signs of insufficient milk supply are when a newborn wants to nurse constantly, cries inconsolably, or is very lethargic, limp, or jaundiced. A baby may also have a reduced number of wet diapers, but this is not a reliable measure because a baby may still produce urine even if they aren't getting enough milk.

The Fed Is Best Foundation also recommends the following steps to prevent and detect hypoglycemia before it becomes a serious problem:

- Manually expressing to confirm the presence of milk
- Twice-daily weighing of exclusively breastfed newborns for the first few days. A weight loss of more than 7% signals the need to supplement with formula.
- Checking blood glucose levels of newborns in the hospital and taking action if the level is below 47 milligrams per deciliter (mg/dL)
- Weighing the baby before and after breastfeeding to determine how much milk is being transferred. Newborns need approximately two ounces every three hours.
- Supplementing with formula after nursing if a baby is crying inconsolably at home, especially before full milk production is established

If you find that you do need to supplement with formula in the first few days after your baby is born, rest assured that this is not likely to undermine your chance of successfully breastfeeding.[30] In Dr. Flaherman's studies demonstrating that point, the following protocol was used: When newborns had lost more weight than usual by their second or third day, mothers were instructed to syringe-feed 10 mL of hypoallergenic formula immediately after each breastfeeding session. The mothers were advised to stop supplementing once their milk supply was established, which typically occurs by around day five.

This strategy has very little downside, but the potential benefits are immense. By ensuring that a baby is getting enough nutrition in the first few days, we can easily prevent low blood sugar and thereby protect the baby's long-term brain health.

The bottom line, according to the Fed Is Best Foundation, is to trust your maternal instincts: "Even brand-new mothers know when something is wrong. Remember that formula feeding is not failure. Fed is best."

Breastfeeding Troubleshooting

If you are planning to breastfeed, learning as much as you can in advance will make it easier to solve any problems that may come up in the first few weeks, when you could be feeling more tired or overwhelmed. Many good resources are available, including La Leche League and lactation consultants. Expert advice in this area can occasionally place too much pressure on breastfeeding while demonizing formula, but you can choose which recommendations to follow and which to ignore. You are the parent, and you have the final say on how to feed your baby.

One of the most common concerns for new breastfeeding mothers is low milk supply. A wide array of products, in the form of supplements, teas, and snack foods, claim to combat this issue. These products typically contain herbs such as fenugreek, fennel, and milk thistle, which have been used in traditional cultures for hundreds of years to increase milk supply. Some evidence indicates that these herbs can have a benefit, albeit a minor one. Fenugreek, for example, may improve milk supply by increasing the production of growth hormone, insulin, and oxytocin.[31] Fennel and milk thistle may also have some benefit, although the scientific research is rather limited. In general, studies indicate that lactation supplements and teas have much less impact than focusing on the major factor governing milk supply: the perceived demand from your baby.

A mother's milk supply is governed by a sophisticated system that responds directly to the baby's needs. Whenever milk is removed from the breast, either by nursing or pumping, this sends a powerful signal to produce more milk. The most effective way to increase your supply is therefore to nurse or pump more often. Studies have found that nursing every two hours instead of three can significantly increase milk production.[32] You can also try pumping after nursing and having longer skin-to-skin contact with your baby each day. The latter is thought to stimulate the release of oxytocin, which encourages the release of milk.

Sometimes when there is a concern about low supply, the real problem is not the mother's ability to produce enough milk but rather the baby's ability to suckle effectively. This is an important side of the equation to address and may require expert help. A good lactation consultant can show you how to optimize the baby's position for better latching and assess whether there may be other potential issues to solve. Nipple shields can also help some babies who have trouble latching.

Clogged Ducts and Mastitis

Another common challenge with breastfeeding is localized pain, typically attributed to clogged ducts or mastitis. Around 20% of nursing mothers develop a firm, painful area of the breast, typically on one side. Once thought to be the result of milk sitting in the ducts for too long and causing blockages, it used to be treated with heat, deep massage, and pumping or hand expressing after feeding to fully empty the breast.

It's now understood that what we think of as "clogged ducts" is most likely part of the spectrum of mastitis, which refers to inflammation of the breast tissue. A reduction in milk flow is more a symptom than a cause. The underlying cause is likely inflammation itself, which narrows the ducts, interfering with the flow of milk and causing painful pressure to build up. With this new understanding, the treatment recommendations have been turned on their head.

In 2022, the Academy of Breastfeeding Medicine issued new guidelines that advise against heat and massage for clogged ducts and localized breast pain while breastfeeding because these treatments can increase inflammation and make the problem worse. Instead, the recommendation is to use ice packs and ibuprofen to reduce swelling and inflammation.[33] This allows the milk ducts to open so milk can flow more freely.

Tylenol can also be used to manage pain, but ibuprofen is more effective in this context because it helps address the underlying inflammation. Ibuprofen is generally considered safe to take while breastfeeding, with only a tiny percentage of the dose being transferred through breast milk, amounting to less than 0.06% of the standard dose of Motrin given to infants to treat pain and fever. [34]

The current guidelines also recommend frequent nursing to relieve pressure but advise against additional pumping after breastfeeding to try to empty the breast and clear the blockage. That is because pumping more milk than your infant needs results in additional milk production, which can cause additional pressure and exacerbate symptoms.[35] The guidelines also suggest feeding first from the unaffected breast to reduce the stimulus for milk production on the affected side.

The Academy of Breastfeeding Medicine also suggests taking a sunflower or soy lecithin supplement. Although not much scientific evidence supports this treatment, there is little downside, and many people find that it helps.

Lecithin is the term for natural fats that can blend oil and water. These fats are found in soybeans, seeds, and egg yolks. Supplementing with lecithin may help clogged ducts and mastitis by reducing inflammation or by emulsifying the fats in milk, thereby reducing the size of fat droplets and allowing milk to flow more freely.

Lecithin also provides a source of choline, although it's difficult to meet your daily choline needs from lecithin alone. A typical dose of sunflower lecithin is two 1,200 milligram capsules, twice per day, for a total of 4,800 milligrams of lecithin. This would provide approximately 100 milligrams of choline. As explained in more detail below, this is far short of the amount needed during breastfeeding.

Breastfeeding Supplements

The supplements that are most helpful when nursing overlap with those recommended during the third trimester, with the highest priorities being choline, calcium, and a multivitamin or prenatal.

Choline is a key ingredient in breast milk because it's needed to support your baby's growth, brain development, detoxification enzymes, and immune function.[36] To keep up with these demands, the recommended daily intake for choline while breastfeeding is at least 550 milligrams per day. To reach this level, you may need to take a standalone choline supplement unless you eat eggs on a daily basis, as covered in Chapter 2.

Another supplement that takes on particular importance during breastfeeding is calcium. A nursing mother likely needs a total of at least 1,200 milligrams per day. Although a dairy-rich diet can help you attain that goal, most women need an extra calcium supplement. The recommended dose is 300–600 milligrams per day. Calcium citrate is the preferred form because it's less likely to cause gastrointestinal side effects than calcium carbonate.

Continuing your daily multivitamin or prenatal while nursing also has value since breastfeeding increases the demand for B vitamins, along with vitamin A, vitamin C, and zinc. To meet these needs, you can continue with your prenatal multivitamin or switch to a general multivitamin. The main difference between the two is that a prenatal typically contains more folate and iron, which can be helpful for replenishing your red blood cells and iron stores after you deliver.

You may also wish to take a fish oil supplement when nursing, but this is optional, and there is limited evidence of its benefit. When it comes to supporting brain development, the research suggests that providing adequate omega-3 fats during the third trimester is far more important. Nevertheless, a higher intake of omega-3 fats when breastfeeding has been linked to lower rates of eczema and allergies in children.[37]

Continuing with a vitamin D supplement is also optional. Doing so can increase the vitamin D content of breast milk, but giving your baby vitamin D drops directly is more reliable.

The American Academy of Pediatrics recommends giving breastfed infants 400 IU per day. The main reason to continue taking vitamin D is to continue supporting your own health and immune system and to promote calcium absorption.

Key Points

- The benefits of breastfeeding over formula feeding are less significant than we're often led to believe, whereas the impact of dehydration and low blood sugar in the first few days of life is often overlooked.

- Some of the purported benefits of breast milk have been exaggerated, but breastfeeding does seem to have a slight edge when it comes to supporting babies' cognitive development and gastrointestinal health.

- To the extent that breastfeeding reduces asthma, allergies, and eczema, this likely occurs by supporting a healthy microbiome, an effect we can mimic with prebiotics and probiotics (see Chapters 19 and 20).

- If milk supply is significantly delayed, newborns can quickly become dehydrated and develop low blood sugar. To avoid this, monitor for sufficient milk supply, such as by weighing your baby before and after initial feedings.

- If your newborn is not getting enough milk, supplementing with formula after nursing can protect their health without undermining breastfeeding success.

Chapter 19

Choosing a Formula

C HOOSING A FORMULA for your baby can feel like a big decision—one that may not be at the forefront of your mind before your baby arrives. But even if you're planning to breastfeed, it can be helpful to have a small supply of formula on hand as you approach your due date, just in case. For this purpose, the initial decision is merely which formula to start with during the first weeks. You may end up switching brands to better meet your baby's needs, or you may find yourself not using any formula if breastfeeding goes well.

During the early weeks, convenience takes on high priority, so it often makes sense to start with a ready-to-feed formula in small bottles. These single servings make life with a newborn much easier because you can typically attach a teat or nipple directly to the bottle and feed right away—without having to prepare powdered formula or wash and sterilize bottles. Good options in the U.S. include Similac 360 Total Care, Enfamil Neuropro, and Enfamil Gentlease. For new parents in the U.K., the best options include Aptamil, Kendamil, and Hipp Organic. Equivalent products exist in most other countries.

There is no clear-cut answer as to which ready-to-feed formula is best to start with, but the major brands are generally good quality, and most babies fare well with any one of the popular options. Babies prone to constipation may feel better with a formula that doesn't contain palm oil, such as Similac 360 Total Care or Kendamil, whereas babies prone to allergies or reflux may have less discomfort with a formula in which the proteins are partially broken down, such as Enfamil Gentlease. It can be a matter of trial and error to see which formula works best for your little one.

If you end up formula feeding beyond the first few weeks and want to choose the best option from among the wider array of powdered formulas, or if your baby seems to be reacting to the formula you started with, you can return to the remainder of this chapter for more in-depth guidance on ingredients to look for and other factors to consider. For those who plan to breastfeed, you can move on to the next chapter, which discusses probiotic and vitamin D supplements for newborns.

Formula Ingredients to Look For

Formula ingredients are heavily regulated and standardized, but there are some differences in the primary proteins, carbohydrates, and fat sources used in different brands. This section will guide you through the preferred options for each component and how to prioritize the factors that matter most.

1. Whey Protein or Partially Hydrolyzed Whey Protein

The single most important factor that determines how well your baby will tolerate a given formula is the type of protein. Cow's-milk formulas are typically a better starting point than soy or goat milk, but even these formulas can differ in the specific types of proteins used.

In both breast milk and cow's milk, the two main types of protein are casein and whey. Breast milk is mostly whey protein, with a smaller amount of casein, whereas the reverse is true for cow's milk, which is 80% casein. The practical difference is that whey is digested much more rapidly. In contrast, casein is more difficult to digest and remains in the stomach for longer. Casein is also considered more "reactive" from an allergy perspective.

To balance out the protein ratio in cow's milk and more closely mimic breast milk, many formula brands now include additional whey protein or use whey as the sole protein source. These formulas typically provide a more suitable starting point for newborns for several reasons. One advantage is that making the formula quicker and easier to digest can reduce spitting up and acid reflux.[1] Whey also produces softer stools, which eases stomach pain for many babies. Finally, a formula with only whey and no whole milk protein will be less allergenic.

If your baby is still not tolerating a whey-based formula, the next step is typically to try one made from partially hydrolyzed whey protein, such as Gerber GentlePro, Similac Total Comfort, or Aptamil Comfort. In these formulas, the whey protein is broken down into shorter pieces, making it easier to digest and less likely to trigger allergies.

Some babies need the proteins to be broken down even more, in the form of an extensively hydrolyzed formula such as Nutramigen. These formulas can have a very unpleasant taste, so many babies don't feed well. They are generally used only when other options have failed.

Other options to consider include soy-based or goat milk formula, which some babies can tolerate better than cow's milk. In the end, no single formula is the best for every baby, and you may need to experiment to find what works for your baby.

2. Lactose as the Primary Carbohydrate Source

The preferred carbohydrate source in baby formula is lactose, as this is the main carbohydrate found in breast milk. Although babies can do well on other carbohydrate sources, such as corn syrup or maltodextrin, it generally makes sense to stay closer to nature when we can.

The main driver behind the use of alternative sugars in baby formula is profit: corn syrup, maltodextrin, and sucrose are much cheaper to produce than lactose. These alternative sugars are also sweeter, which increases the chance that a baby will willingly take a new formula.

Some companies may use corn syrup or other sugars in order to cater to parents' concerns over lactose intolerance. Yet very few babies have genuine difficulty with lactose.[2] It's far more common for a baby to react to the protein component in formula. In studies of babies with colic, switching to a lactose-free formula can occasionally help, but it often makes little difference.[3]

A better strategy for dealing with colic is to choose a partially hydrolyzed whey formula containing prebiotics and to supplement with probiotics, as discussed in more detail in Chapter 19. A formula containing lactose is more likely to help babies build a healthy microbiome, which may prevent colic.[4]

Although our starting point should be choosing a formula that contains lactose as the main carbohydrate source, no specific evidence exists that corn syrup, maltodextrin, or other sugars in formula are harmful. Corn syrup and maltodextrin are easily digestible forms of glucose produced by breaking down cornstarch. In hydrolyzed formulas in particular, these other sugars may be needed to disguise the bitter taste from the broken-down proteins.

Corn syrup and maltodextrin may sound like poor choices for your baby's nutrition, but they're safe ingredients and are much better than sucrose, which contains a high proportion of fructose. Babies have difficulty metabolizing fructose, and large amounts of this sugar could place an unnecessary burden on the liver. For this reason, it's best to avoid formulas that list sucrose early in the ingredients unless it's needed for your baby to willingly take a hypoallergenic formula.

If a formula meets all your other requirements but contains corn syrup or maltodextrin as the carbohydrate, this should not be a deal-breaker. It's just preferable to have lactose as the main carbohydrate to more closely approximate breast milk.

2. Prebiotics

Prebiotics are indigestible carbohydrates that serve to nourish beneficial gut microbes. Breast milk contains hundreds of different prebiotics in quite large amounts. Collectively, these prebiotics are known as human milk oligosaccharides (HMOs).

The HMOs in breast milk seem to be tailor-made to feed only beneficial species, such as *Bifidobacteria*. This is thought to be the main reason breastfed babies seem to have a healthier balance of species in their gut microbiome.

In recent years, formula manufacturers have developed strategies to mimic this extraordinary property by adding various prebiotics in an effort to nourish the beneficial bacteria. The evidence shows that this strategy is quite effective when it comes to building a healthier microbiome in formula-fed babies.[5]

One of the first prebiotics to be introduced to infant formula is known as GOS, which stands for galactooligosaccharides. Research has shown that babies receiving formula containing GOS develop similar levels of beneficial microbes as breastfed infants.[6]

Infant formulas supplemented with a combination of GOS and another type of prebiotic, fructooligosaccharides (FOS), have also been studied in numerous randomized, double-blind, placebo-controlled studies, with very promising results.[7]

These studies indicate that giving prebiotics to formula-fed infants significantly lowers the risk of respiratory and gastrointestinal infections as well as allergic conditions such as asthma and eczema.[8] In one study in which infants were given breast milk, prebiotic formula, or standard formula, the prebiotic formula was found to reduce the risk of food allergy in much the same way as breast milk.[9] Seventeen percent of children in the standard formula group had food allergies by 18 months, compared to just 4% of breastfed infants and 5% of infants given the prebiotic formula.

After reviewing all the studies in this area, the World Allergy Organization recently issued guidelines recommending prebiotic supplementation for formula-fed infants to reduce the risk of developing asthma, eczema, and food allergy.[10]

In just the past few years, formula makers have found a way to mimic the prebiotics found in breast milk even more closely by adding a lactose derivative known as 2'-fucosyllactose (2'-FL). This is the most abundant prebiotic in breast milk. It can now be produced in the laboratory by fermentation (similar to how many vitamins are made), resulting in a prebiotic that is structurally identical to that found in breast milk. Several studies have demonstrated that including this important prebiotic in formula can improve the balance of gut bacteria in young babies, resulting in a higher proportion of beneficial species and fewer harmful species.[11]

This prebiotic is now included in several premium formula brands, where it is listed in the ingredients as 2'-FL HMO (Human Milk Oligosaccharide). At the time of writing, formulas containing this prebiotic include:

- Enfamil NeuroPro
- Gerber Good Start Soothe Pro
- Gerber Good Start Gentle Pro
- Similac 360 Total Care
- Similac Pro-Total Comfort
- Kirkland Signature Pro Care
- Store brand Advantage Premium
- Store brand Infant Premium

Another prebiotic found naturally in breast milk and now added to formula is a combination of galactose and lactose known as 3'-GL. This prebiotic is found in Kendamil Infant formula and Kendamil Organic formula and can likely support the development of a healthy microbiome in much the same way as other prebiotics.

3. Milk Fat Globule Membrane (MFGM)

One of the most perplexing issues facing formula manufacturers is the slight edge breastfed children have on IQ and vocabulary tests. The difference in scores is relatively minor once you control for the other factors that typically go along with breastfeeding, such as higher IQ and education level among nursing mothers, but there is still a gap.[12] This suggests some additional component is present in breast milk that plays a role in brain development.

In just the past few years, research has pointed to the possibility that this component is found in the thin layer surrounding fat globules in breast milk, known as milk fat globule membrane, or MFGM for short. This collection of various proteins and lipids, including several components needed for the production of new brain cells, is present in much higher amounts in breast milk than cow's milk. When formula is made by using purified cow's milk proteins while obtaining fats from other sources, most of the MFGM is left behind.

To address this problem, researchers developed a method to isolate pure MFGM from cow's milk so it can be added to formula. Several studies have now reported encouraging results with this approach, including cognitive scores similar to breastfed babies.[13] One such study followed up with the children years later and found that the benefits are no longer evident on IQ tests once children reach six years old. However, an IQ test is a fairly narrow measure of brain function, and other benefits may persist.[14] Studies have also found that MFGM helps protect against harmful microbes and intestinal inflammation, likely reducing the chance of colic.[15]

To take advantage of these potential benefits, a number of formulas are now marketed as containing MFGM, including:

- Enfamil NeuroPro
- Enfamil Enspire
- Kendamil Infant Formula
- Kendamil Organic
- Aussie Bubs
- Generic equivalents of Enfamil NeuroPro

We don't yet know whether these formulas contain enough MFGM to truly make a difference. The studies in this area typically looked at formulas with purified MFGM added as a separate ingredient, whereas the formulas that are commercially available rely on the presence of MFGM in other ingredients.

Enfamil and its generic equivalents are labeled as containing "naturally occurring MFGM components from whey protein concentrate." An independent study by researchers in New Zealand and the University of California investigating various commercial sources of MFGM found that Enfamil Enspire does contain more MFGM than standard Enfamil formula.[16] It also contains more of the specific lipids likely to be involved in brain development. This indicates that Enfamil's manufacturer is processing the whey protein differently to preserve more MFGM in their premium formula versions, although whether the amount is enough to make a practical difference is unproven.

Enfamil Enspire has the added benefit of lactoferrin, one of the whey proteins found in breast milk that helps fight off harmful microbes. Standard formula already contains some lactoferrin, so this is not a critical ingredient, but the higher concentration in Enfamil Enspire may provide added defense against gastrointestinal infections.[17]

It remains unclear whether the store brand versions of Enfamil NeuroPro also contain higher amounts of MFGM than other formulas or whether their labeling is relying on the small amount of MFGM naturally present in standard whey protein concentrate.

Kendamil takes a slightly different approach and relies on the MFGM naturally present in milk fat. Rather than taking only the purified proteins from cow's milk and then adding fats such as palm oil and safflower oil, the first ingredient in Kendamil is whole milk, which should contain some MFGM within the milk fat component. Little data is available on how much MFGM is in Kendamil, but it is likely significantly more than in standard formula. The Aussie Bubs formula also contains whole milk powder to provide a source of MFGM, although it's lower on the list of ingredients than in Kendamil.

Overall, choosing a formula higher in MFMG is probably helpful for supporting brain development during the early months, particularly if you are exclusively formula feeding. This is a lower priority if you're merely supplementing with formula or have previously breastfed and are now switching to formula. In those cases, your baby has likely been getting a good supply of MFGM while nursing. MFGM is also a lower priority once your baby starts solids at four to six months. At that point, you can provide other sources of milk fat, such as butter, cream, or full-fat yogurt.

4. Fats and Oils

Most formulas include a combination of safflower, palm, soy, and coconut oils to replicate the range of fats present in breast milk. All serve as good fat sources for babies, and the precise combination of oils typically makes little difference. The one factor that may impact how well your baby tolerates a formula is the amount of palm oil.

Palm oil is often used as a primary fat source in formula because of its high concentration of palmitic acid, which is also found in large amounts in breast milk. The potential downside to palm oil is that the fats are present in a form that can bind to calcium and cause constipation in some babies. If your baby seems uncomfortable, you may consider trying a formula without palm oil, such as one of the Similac varieties, Kendamil, or Kirkland Pro Care.

For most babies, however, the type of oil present shouldn't be a major consideration in choosing a formula. Instead, it's more important to look for some or all of the preferred ingredients discussed earlier, especially prebiotics.

Organic, European, and Generic Formulas

One pitfall of prioritizing the newer specialty formula ingredients is that finding a formula that's also organic becomes more difficult. Many parents would prefer an organic formula due to concerns about traces of pesticides or antibiotics.

The drawback is that prioritizing an organic formula narrows the options significantly. This is especially true if your baby has reflux or colic and you need a partially hydrolyzed or whey-only formula.

Deciding between organic and nonorganic is ultimately a matter of personal preference and weighing priorities, but the current data suggests it's more important to focus on giving your baby beneficial nutrients such as prebiotics. Even if pesticides are present in conventional milk, that doesn't necessarily mean they'll find their way into infant formula made from that milk, given the degree of processing that occurs. If a formula manufacturer takes only highly purified whey protein and lactose from milk, the pesticides and other contaminants are largely left behind.

In one study of more than 300 samples of conventional milk and infant formulas, pesticide residues were detected in the milk but not in the formulas.[18] Other researchers have either reported the same result or have found extremely low levels of pesticides in only a small minority of formulas.[19]

Overall, the risk of exposure to pesticides from standard formula is very low and on a par with breast milk, given that mothers consume pesticides through food and pass it on to their baby via breastfeeding. One study found that the level of pesticide residues was *higher* in human breast milk than in conventional formula.[20]

All of this suggests that it's not crucial to choose an organic formula and that we should instead prioritize beneficial ingredients such as prebiotics.

Another common question among parents in the United States is whether formulas imported from Europe may be higher quality or have safer ingredients. The idea that European formulas are superior has some intuitive appeal, given the lax regulation of other products in the United States. A vast array of chemicals that are banned in Europe are found in everything from sunscreen to potato chips in America. But the same pattern does not apply to infant formula. Formula is strictly regulated, and there is little reason to be concerned about the safety or quality of ingredients in American infant formulas, whether they are premium or generic brands.

Generic formulas are a good option, especially if you're on a tight budget. In the United States, these formulas are sold under various store brands, but they're made by a single manufacturer. Whether you buy the store brand associated with Target, Walmart, Sam's Club, Kroger, or Amazon, all are made by Perrigo and contain exactly the same ingredients across the different store brands. Each specific generic formula is intended to closely correspond to a particular Enfamil or Similac formula.

For example, the Infant Premium formula sold under Walmart's store brand is identical to the Infant Premium formula at Target. This particular formula is intended to replicate the ingredients in Enfamil NeuroPro. Similarly, each store brand's Advantage Premium formula is intended to replicate

Similac 360 Total Care. Kirkland's ProCare infant formula is also made by Perrigo and is another Similac equivalent.

In some cases, minor differences in ingredients may exist between the name-brand and store-brand formulas, and it's not clear how well Perrigo has been able to replicate the MFGM found in Enfamil, but overall, the quality should be closely comparable.

Preparing Formula

One point on which experts disagree is whether it's necessary to sterilize infant formula during the first two months. The purpose of doing so is to eliminate the microbe *Cronobacter*, which can survive in dry ingredients such as powdered formula and can cause serious infections in newborns. These infections are incredibly rare, with around one or two cases reported to the CDC each year. Extensive testing and monitoring for *Cronobacter* also occurs at formula manufacturing facilities, so the chance of the microbe coming from formula rather than the general environment is low.

Even so, the CDC recommends that for babies who are younger than two months, born prematurely, or who have a weakened immune system, it's safest to sterilize powdered formula. This can be done by preparing the formula with hot water above 160° F (70° C). The temperature does not have to be exact; the CDC simply recommends boiling water, allowing it to cool for five minutes, then mixing with the powdered formula.

The simplest way to do this is usually to gather a batch of bottles for the day, pour the correct amount of water into each bottle from an electric tea kettle, add the powder, and then store the prepared formula in the refrigerator until needed. This procedure is not necessary for ready-to-feed liquid formula, which is already sterilized.

When bottle feeding at home, choosing glass baby bottles over plastic is recommended to avoid potential exposure to chemicals, even in BPA-free plastic. Glass also stays cleaner and can be washed in the dishwasher. If you're sending your baby to a daycare where glass is not allowed, the next best option is stainless steel, but this is usually only practical if your baby will happily take refrigerator-temperature milk or if the daycare heats milk in bottle warmers rather than the microwave. Otherwise, the next best option is to use bottles made from polypropylene or silicone.

How Much Formula Does a Baby Need?

First days	1 to 2 ounces per bottle every 2 to 3 hours
First weeks	2 to 3 ounces per bottle every 3 to 4 hours
1 month old	3 to 4 ounces per bottle every 3 to 4 hours
2 months old	4 to 5 ounces per bottle every 3 to 4 hours
3 months old	4 to 6 ounces per bottle every 3 to 4 hours
4 months old	4 to 6 ounces per bottle, 4 to 6 times a day
6 months old	6 to 8 ounces per bottle, 4 to 5 times a day

Key Points

- To more closely replicate breast milk, look for a formula that contains:
- whey protein or partially hydrolyzed whey
- lactose as the primary carbohydrate
- prebiotics such as GOS or 2'-FL
- milk fat globule membrane (MFGM)
- Choosing a formula with optimal ingredients is generally more important than buying organic since infant formula has been found to have little or no pesticide residues.
- For babies with allergies, colic, or reflux, a partially hydrolyzed, 100% whey-based formula is usually the best option.
- For babies with constipation, choosing a formula without palm oil can be helpful.

Chapter 20

Newborn Probiotics and Vitamin D

ONE OF THE most important jobs a newborn baby has is developing an internal ecosystem of beneficial gut microbes. This process occurs throughout the body but takes on greater importance in the gastrointestinal tract. There, bacteria help process milk, synthesize vitamins, regulate the immune system, and prevent infection.

These microbes are so important that by adulthood, the number of beneficial bacteria in the gut will outnumber all the human cells in the entire body—by a factor of 10 to 1. In newborns, however, this important ecosystem has not yet been established, so the gut microbiome is more or less a blank slate.[1]

After babies are born, they must build their own microbiome from the ground up. They will typically acquire some bacteria from the birth canal during vaginal birth, but most species are collected over the subsequent days and weeks through breast milk, contact with parents, and the general environment.

If you delivered by C-section, had antibiotics during labor, or are exclusively formula feeding, this normal process may be compromised to some extent, with fewer beneficial microbes and a greater proportion of unwanted species.[2] Giving your baby probiotics during the first few weeks may help address this imbalance, supporting the development of a healthy microbiome.

For babies without any factors impairing the transfer of beneficial microbes, probiotics may be considered more of an optional extra, but they're probably beneficial if you have a family history of allergies, asthma, or eczema. Certain probiotics may also help prevent and manage colic and reflux.

Overcoming Modern Threats to the Microbiome

Although C-sections, antibiotics during delivery, and formula feeding typically get most of the blame when it comes to disruptions to the microbiome, a baby may also lack important microbes simply by virtue of living in the modern world.

Over the last century, a general loss of certain beneficial species has occurred in the population of developed countries. Researchers have found that in typical U.S. communities, more than 90% of infants are lacking *Bifidobacterium infantis*, a species that appears to be particularly important in newborn babies.[3]

Interest in this species was sparked when researchers discovered that it's much better at metabolizing the prebiotics found in breast milk than all other species.[4] In other words, breast milk seems to be tailor-made to encourage *B. infantis* to thrive. This suggests that humans evolved alongside *B. infantis*, likely with major benefits for a baby's health.

One of these benefits is protection from harmful microbes.[5] As Professor Bruce German of the University of California explains, "The central benefit of having a microbiota dominated by *B. infantis* is that it crowds all the other guys out— especially pathogenic bacteria, which can cause both acute illnesses and chronic inflammation that leads to disease." As a result, *B. infantis* has been found to significantly reduce the risk of serious infections in premature babies.[6]

Another important benefit of having enough bifidobacteria during infancy is education and training of the immune system. As explained by Dr. Katri Korpela, an immunobiologist at the University of Helsinki, "The immune system is constantly talking with the microbes in the gut." Beneficial microbes help set the dial on the immune system, a process that is particularly critical during infancy, when the long-term programming of the immune system happens. Without this education, the immune system may be more likely to overreact to food allergens, for example.

In recent decades, babies in the developed world have begun to lose these benefits of bifidobacteria, with most babies no longer being colonized with *B. infantis*.[7] Formula feeding and C-sections may play a role in this decline, but since this species is lacking even in many breastfed babies delivered by vaginal birth, the main culprit is likely the general loss of the species in the modern population. If mothers don't have this microbe to begin with, it can't be passed down to their babies.

In countries in the developing world, such as Gambia and Bangladesh, *B. infantis* is still the dominant species in new babies.[8] It's also one of the dominant species in Old Order

Mennonites in the United States. When researchers recently studied infants in one of these traditional rural farming communities, they found that more than 70% of babies still carried *B. infantis*.[9]

Giving a newborn baby a probiotic containing *B. infantis* may help restore this natural state of affairs. This could in turn reduce some of the afflictions that are overrepresented in the developed world, such as food allergies, asthma, eczema, and autoimmune conditions.[10] In the study of Old Order Mennonites, less than 7% of the Mennonite children went on to develop allergies, asthma, or eczema, compared to 35% of matched children in a nearby suburban community.

A variety of probiotics formulated for babies now contain *B. infantis*, including Evivo's infant probiotic and LoveBug's baby probiotic drops. For additional recommendations, see itstartswiththebump.com/infant-probiotics.

B. infantis is likely one of the best probiotic strains for newborns, but it's far from the only choice. Other bifidobacteria species and a lactobacillus species known as *L. rhamnosus* GG (LGG) appear to produce many similar benefits, including reducing the negative impact of antibiotics and C-sections, suppressing pathogens, and calibrating the immune system to prevent allergies.[11]

Another probiotic strain that has been extensively studied in newborn babies is *L. reuteri* DSM 17938. Originally obtained from the breast milk of a Peruvian mother, this strain is sold as BioGaia Protectis and Gerber Soothe probiotic drops. The key strength of *L. reuteri* lies in its ability to combat harmful microbes. For this reason, many hospitals give this probiotic to premature babies in the NICU to prevent serious gastrointestinal infections, likely saving countless lives.[12] It's also very effective at combatting stomach bugs in older children.[13]

Probiotics can inhibit harmful species in two ways. First, the probiotic strains of bacteria take up real estate and compete for nutrients, providing less opportunity for harmful species to flourish. This is one of the main advantages of building a good population of bifidobacteria species. Second, certain probiotic strains, such as *L. rhamnosus* and *L. reuteri*, produce powerful antimicrobial compounds to directly target and suppress pathogens while leaving other beneficial species unharmed.[14] The combination of probiotics that serve both functions is likely to be particularly helpful for new babies so they can develop a diverse population of beneficial microbes without disruption from harmful species.

Probiotic Timing

The most useful time to give probiotics is in the first few weeks, when your baby is first establishing a community of microbes and has little resistance to harmful species. Once you have successfully seeded their microbiome with beneficial bacteria, much of the work is done. That means it's generally not necessary to continue probiotics beyond the first one or two months.

There may be further need for probiotics if your baby receives antibiotics, experiences digestive issues, or develops colic or reflux. As the following sections explain, in such scenarios, it's useful to continue with a probiotic such as *B. infantis* while also incorporating a specific strain that can help tackle the situation at hand.

Continuing probiotics beyond the first months is also recommended if your baby shows signs of allergies or eczema and needs the additional help to calm their immune system. The strains most likely to be helpful for this purpose are *L. rhamnosus* GG (LGG) and *B. infantis*.

Probiotics for Colic

Babies with colic typically cry for many hours a day, for reasons that long remained a mystery. With the advent of new technology to analyze the microbiome, researchers have been able to see distinct differences in the gut bacteria of these infants.

It's now believed that colic is often caused by abdominal pain due to an excess of inflammatory bacteria.[15] By suppressing these harmful species and calming the inflammation, probiotics can prevent or alleviate colic for many babies. This has recently been demonstrated in several clinical trials, with particularly good evidence for *L. reuteri* DSM 17938. This probiotic significantly reduces crying time in babies with colic, while also reducing markers of gut inflammation.[16]

Probiotics are not always a quick fix because it can take several weeks for your baby's microbiome to rebalance, but persistence often pays off. One study found that after 30 days, babies given *L. reuteri* DSM 17938 cried for half as much time each day as babies in the placebo group.[17]

B. infantis may also help prevent or treat colic, although this has not been studied as extensively in this context as *L. reuteri* DSM 17938. What we do know is that *B. infantis* reduces intestinal inflammation in newborns, and on average, the more bifidobacteria babies have, the less they cry during the first three months.[18]

If you have a colicky baby, they could benefit from both of these probiotics to tackle the problem from multiple angles. If your goal is merely prevention, one option is to start with *B. infantis* and then add *L. reuteri* DSM 17938 later if needed.

Probiotics for Reflux

For some babies who cry for many hours each day, the issue may not be typical colic but rather acid reflux. Spitting up milk several times per day is very common among young babies and not normally an issue, but in rare cases the acidic stomach contents can irritate a baby's esophagus, causing near-constant discomfort. These babies often spit up much more than normal and cry intensely for many hours every day, particularly after feeding.

If your baby has reflux, it's often a matter of making it through the difficult early months, waiting for their stomach to mature. Most babies outgrow the problem at around four months, when the muscle that separates the stomach and esophagus starts to work more effectively. In the meantime, probiotics may help reduce the severity of symptoms.

The strain most likely to be helpful is again *L. reuteri* DSM-17938. The reason it's so effective for reflux is not well understood, but studies have found that it can reduce the number of episodes of spitting up, increase the speed at which the stomach empties, increase the frequency of bowel movements, and significantly reduce crying time.[19]

If you are formula feeding, studies also indicate that a starch-thickened formula made with partially hydrolyzed whey protein can help. When given in combination with the *L. reuteri* probiotic, this type of formula reduced the average number of regurgitations from more than seven times per day to fewer than three,[20] an improvement that could significantly reduce the irritation of the esophagus and eventually lessen a baby's discomfort.

The Holistic Approach to Colic and Reflux

by Dr. Elisa Song, M.D., author of *Healthy Kids, Happy Kids: An Integrative Pediatrician's Guide to Whole Child Resilience*

When I graduated from my pediatrics residency in 2000, it was unheard of to use antacids in babies. Just a few years later, Zantac was approved for infants and suddenly became a common treatment for fussiness and colic, based on the theory that the babies were in pain due to acid reflux.

In 2018, the tide began to shift again, with a study of almost 800,000 infants finding that early use of antacids doubled the risk of food allergy.[21] Dr. Edward Mitre, who led this study, commented that "antibiotics and antacids might change the makeup of a baby's microbiome, perhaps enough to cause an overreaction in the immune system that shows up as an allergy."

In light of this study, pediatricians now prescribe antacids more judiciously and look for other approaches to help babies with abdominal pain and colic. Luckily, there are so many other things we can do from an integrative and functional medicine standpoint.

The first thing to realize is that for most babies, reflux or colic is caused by inflammation in their gut. Often this is due to an imbalance in gut bacteria, so I recommend giving babies probiotics, specifically *L. reuteri* and an infant probiotic combination.

In other cases, babies have gut inflammation because they are reacting to either their formula or something in breast milk. For formula-fed babies, a partially hydrolyzed or hypoallergenic formula may help. For babies who are breastfeeding, I typically have moms follow an elimination diet for two weeks to exclude some of the biggest culprits, such as dairy, gluten, soy, eggs, and citrus. If you take out all those foods, many babies are much better within just a few days. We can then add the foods back one by one and see how the baby responds.

Herbal medicine can also be helpful. Many years ago, a study found that herbs such as chamomile, ginger, lemon balm, and fennel seed can help relieve colic symptoms.[22] These herbs are included in gripe water, which can be quite effective in calming a baby's digestive system.

If all these measures fail and a baby is still spitting up constantly, arching their back, and screaming after feedings, they may have reflux caused by an immature valve that keeps milk in the stomach. In these cases, feeding babies smaller amounts less often, with frequent burping during feedings, can be helpful. Holding your baby upright for half an hour after feedings can also reduce their symptoms. If your baby is still in great discomfort after all these measures, we might then consider an antacid as a last resort.

We also have to remember that sometimes fussiness is just a side effect of normal brain development. Starting at around two weeks old, babies begin to spend more time awake and become more aware of their surroundings. It's normal for babies to go through a fussy period at this time, with sensory overload from the day causing them to cry more than normal, particularly in the early evenings. This usually peaks at around 6–8 weeks, then improves as the baby's brain starts to mature and the social smile starts to develop, and babies are able to take in the world without getting overstimulated. Once the fussy stage passes, life gets better. If your baby is still in this difficult phase, understand that this is normal and use soothing and comforting techniques until it passes.

When your baby is miserable, it's natural to want to solve the problem as quickly as possible by going straight to medication. But now that we know antacids can have long-term impacts on a baby's immune system, and even the developing brain, it makes sense to try other strategies first. The holistic, functional medicine approach to colic and reflux is a process, not a quick fix, but it will help your baby thrive so much better in the long run.

Bouncing Back from Antibiotics

It's understandable to feel a little disappointed if your baby needs antibiotics, as this can be a setback to cultivating a healthy gut microbiome. Perhaps unsurprisingly, children who receive multiple courses of antibiotics in the early years are more likely to develop asthma, eczema, and food allergies.[23]

The good news is that if your child does need antibiotics, you may be able to significantly reduce the negative impact by supplementing with probiotics. The right strains can reduce the disruption to the microbiome and help the population of beneficial microbes recover sooner.[24]

In clinical studies, the two probiotics found to have the most impact in this context are *S. boulardii* and LGG.[25] When given in combination with antibiotics, both prevent harmful species such as *E. coli* and yeasts from taking hold.[26] They also help the microbiome recover more rapidly after antibiotic treatment ends, allowing other beneficial species to bounce back.[27] In addition, both *S. boulardii* and LGG have a long track record of safety in clinical studies, including in newborn babies.[28] Other probiotics strains you may already have on hand, such as *B. infantis* or *L. reuteri,* can also help protect your baby's microbiome. The main goal of probiotics during and after antibiotic treatment is to take up real estate and suppress harmful yeasts and bacteria until the population of beneficial microbes rebounds.

Boosting the Immune System with Vitamin D

Supporting your child's natural immunity against infections can also help in avoiding the potential harms of antibiotics, as Dr. Song explains: "In my practice, I focus on boosting children's immune systems throughout the year to reduce the chance of any illness requiring antibiotics. One important element of this is maintaining good vitamin D levels."

Studies have shown that children with adequate levels of vitamin D have significantly lower rates of infection. As one example, pediatricians in Japan performed a randomized, double-blind study where they gave children vitamin D supplements throughout the winter and tracked the number of cases of influenza. In the vitamin D–supplemented group, just 11% developed flu, compared to 19% in the placebo group.[29] Such a clear reduction in infections is useful in itself but likely has the additional benefit of reducing the need for antibiotics. That is because congestion caused by viruses can often lead to secondary bacterial infections such as pneumonia, bronchitis, or ear infections, which may end up requiring antibiotics.

Preventing infections is one of the greatest benefits of ensuring that your baby gets enough vitamin D, but it's not the only one. Vitamin D is also critical to bone health, and babies with adequate vitamin D show improved growth and stronger bones.[30] Avoiding a vitamin D deficiency in infancy may also lower the risk of developing asthma, eczema, and allergies.[31]

Given these important benefits, it's troubling that many babies still don't get an adequate amount. One study in Boston found that 40% of babies had suboptimal levels.[32] This widespread problem is recognized by the American Academy of Pediatrics (AAP), which recommends giving babies supplemental vitamin D starting soon after birth.

Initially, the AAP's recommendation applied only to breastfed babies since it was thought that formula-fed infants were already getting enough vitamin D from the amount added to formula. But in 2010, researchers at the Centers for Disease Control (CDC) found that only a third of exclusively formula-fed babies were drinking enough formula each day to meet their vitamin D needs.[33] The CDC researchers concluded that "most infants, not just those who are breastfed, may require an oral vitamin D supplement daily, beginning within their first few days of life."

The AAP's current recommendation states:

Pediatricians should encourage parents of infants who are either breastfed or consuming less than 1 liter (just under 1 quart, or 33.8 ounces) of infant formula per day to give their infants an oral vitamin D supplement.[34]

The dose recommended by the AAP is 400 IU per day, which is typically one drop of an infant vitamin D supplement. Some infant probiotics, such as BioGaia Protectis, already contain this amount, so separate vitamin D drops may not be needed.

The vitamin D supplement should be continued until your little one can get sufficient amounts from other sources, typically through brief daily sun exposure once they are at least six months old, or when they are regularly eating vitamin D–rich food, such as salmon. In colder climates, many children continue to need a vitamin D supplement throughout the winter.

If you are primarily breastfeeding, an alternative to giving your baby daily vitamin D drops is taking a higher dose your-self. To achieve adequate levels in breast milk, you would likely need to take at least 6,000 IU per day.[35] This can be more con-venient and gives you the many benefits of vitamin D, too, but it's a less reliable method than giving vitamin D to babies directly. Different individuals absorb and process vitamin D differently, so the amount transferred in breast milk can be unpredictable. One solution is to take 5,000 IU per day your-self and also give your baby vitamin D drops several times per week to make sure they are getting enough.

Key Points

- Babies in modern populations are missing key microbes that help process milk, regulate the immune system, and outcompete harmful bacteria.

- Probiotics such as *B. infantis* can help fill this gap, potentially reducing the chance of colic, gastrointestinal infections, asthma, eczema, and food allergies.

- The most important time for probiotics is in the early weeks when your baby is first establishing their microbiome.

- Continuing probiotics longer may be helpful to manage colic and reflux. One of the most useful strains for this purpose is *L. reuteri* DSM 17938, found in BioGaia Protectis infant drops.

- Giving your baby a vitamin D supplement can help support their growth and immune system. The recommended dose is 400 IU per day.

Epilogue

OVER THE TEN years since *It Starts with the Egg* was first published, the single most common question I get from readers is one I'm always happy to see:

I just got a positive pregnancy test! What supplements should I stop and what do I need to add?

This question often arises at an overwhelming moment. Someone may have waited years to see those two pink lines for the first time or may have seen them before but worry about what comes next.

When I originally set out to write this book, my goal was to answer questions about supplements and other topics that are high priorities for those who are pregnant after a struggle with infertility or miscarriage. There are a few unique considerations in these situations, given that age, IVF, and other factors can sometimes impact the placenta and increase the odds of complications. Yet as I began investigating these issues, it became clear that the most important strategies for preventing complications and having a healthy pregnancy are relevant for *all* pregnancies, regardless of whether reaching this point was easy or difficult. It also became clear that much of this information wasn't reaching people in time, since conventional medicine often focuses on diagnosis and treatment rather than prevention.

Once you've experienced firsthand the impact of going beyond the standard advice and acting on the latest scientific research, it becomes difficult to go back to passively accepting the conventional wisdom. There is a much stronger desire to be well informed and to do everything you can to improve the odds, right from the start.

That is ultimately what this book is about. As I delved into the scientific research, I found a wide array of discoveries that can improve the odds of having a healthy pregnancy but have not yet filtered down into standard practice. Fortunately, we can put these discoveries into practice now, rather than waiting for the world to catch up. By doing so, it becomes possible to reduce the chance of pregnancy complications, have an easier labor and postpartum recovery, and support a baby's growth, immune system, and brain development.

Whatever brought you to this book, I hope you now feel more confident and informed, knowing you're acting on the latest evidence to support your health and your baby's health during this extraordinary time.

I extend my deepest gratitude to everyone who has shared their stories and questions over the years and to the scientists and medical researchers who made this book possible. The strategies in these chapters represent the life's work of thousands of scientists dedicated to improving maternal and infant health. Please join me in spreading the word about their important findings by sharing this book with anyone who might find it useful.

Timeline for a Proactive Pregnancy

First Trimester (Weeks 1-12)

- Have your thyroid hormones tested as soon as possible; ferritin should be tested at your first prenatal checkup
- Start taking a prenatal, choline, vitamin D, omega-3, and optionally calcium (calcium can be started in the second trimester if preferred).
- Consider adding CoQ10 and NAC if you have a history of miscarriage;
- Consider starting myo-inositol if you have risk factors for gestational diabetes (or postpone until second trimester or glucose tolerance test)
- Complete NIPT screening at 10–12 weeks if you plan to do this testing
- Start core stability exercises if you feel up to it

Second Trimester (Weeks 13-27)

- Continue prenatal, choline, vitamin D, and omega 3
- Start taking calcium if not already
- Start myo-inositol if you have significant risk factors for gestational diabetes or your glucose tolerance test suggests insulin resistance
- Add on low-dose aspirin if you have risk factors for preeclampsia (this is taken during weeks 12–24)

Third Trimester (Weeks 28–40)

- Continue prenatal, choline, vitamin D, omega-3, and calcium

- Continue myo-inositol if taking.

- Consider taking additional iron

- Stop omega-3 supplement at 36 weeks

- Consider receiving the Tdap vaccine at 28–32 weeks and RSV vaccine at 32–36 weeks; Flu and COVID vaccine timing is typically according to viral season

- See a pelvic floor physical therapist or start breathing exercises and pelvic floor stretches at approximately 35 weeks to prepare for labor

Postpartum/ Breastfeeding

- Continue taking your prenatal, choline, and calcium

- Omega-3 and vitamin D are likely beneficial but not essential

- Continue or increase iron for at least a month after delivery to replenish your iron stores

- Give your baby vitamin D drops until they can obtain enough vitamin D from sun exposure and food

- Give your baby probiotic drops during the first month to establish a robust microbiome; continue if needed to address colic or reflux

Supplement Overview

Core supplements

Prenatal

- Look for a brand containing methylfolate (rather than synthetic folic acid) plus the complete spectrum of B vitamins and, ideally, iron in the form of iron bisglycinate.

Choline

- To support your baby's brain development, aim for 450–550 milligrams per day of choline from food and supplements.
- You can likely reach this target by eating two or three eggs most days or taking a supplementing providing around 350 milligrams.

Omega-3 fish oil

- To reduce the odds of preterm birth, take a supplement containing between 500 and 1,000 milligrams of omega-3 fats with at least 500 milligrams of DHA or eat salmon or sardines at least twice per week.
- Omega-3 supplements should be stopped at 36 weeks.

Vitamin D

- The optimal level of vitamin D during pregnancy is at least 40 ng/mL (or 100 nmol/L).
- Most people need to supplement with at least 4,000 IU per day to reach that target.

Calcium

- Getting enough calcium in the second and third trimesters helps protect your bone health and prevent preeclampsia.
- Most people need to supplement with 400–600 milligrams of calcium per day.
- Combining calcium with magnesium is optional, but it may help manage common pregnancy symptoms such as insomnia, constipation, muscle pain, and headaches.

Iron

- The recommended minimum intake in pregnancy is 27 milligrams per day, but some people may need 40 milligrams or more per day to address anemia.
- If your prenatal contains very little iron, if you're vegetarian, or if your ferritin is low, you may need to add a separate iron supplement, particularly when iron needs increase in the second and third trimesters.
- The best forms are iron bisglycinate and heme iron polypeptide.

Add-ons for specific situations

CoQ10 and NAC

- If you have experienced miscarriages in the past and suspect immune or blood-clotting issues, consider taking 200 milligrams of CoQ10 and 600 milligrams of NAC, at least during the first trimester.

Myo-inositol

- If you have PCOS, a higher BMI, or a history of gestational diabetes, consider taking myo-inositol to manage your blood sugar. It is most useful in the second trimester but can be started at any time.
- Myo-inositol may also be worthwhile if you're of Asian descent or have higher odds of developing gestational diabetes due to your age.
- The typical dose is 4 grams per day, half in the morning and half at night.

Aspirin

- If you're over 35, conceived by IVF, or have another risk factor for preeclampsia, consider taking low-dose aspirin from weeks 12 through 24.
- The recommended dose is 80–160 milligrams per day, which is typically one or two low-dose aspirin tablets.
- If you do develop preeclampsia, L-arginine may help manage your blood pressure. A typical dose is 3 grams per day.

References

Chapter 1. Choosing the Best Prenatal Supplement

1   Crider, K. S., Devine, O., Hao, L., Dowling, N. F., Li, S., Molloy, A. M., ... & Berry, R. J. (2014). Population red blood cell folate concentrations for prevention of neural tube defects: Bayesian model. Bmj, 349.
    Daly LE, Kirke PN, Molloy A, Weir DG, Scott JM. Folate levels and neural tube defects. Implications for prevention. JAMA. 1995;274:1698–702.
2   Fazili, Z., Paladugula, N., Zhang, M., & Pfeiffer, C. M. (2021). Folate forms in red blood cell lysates and conventionally prepared whole blood lysates appear stable for up to 2 years at– 70° C and show comparable concentrations. *The Journal of Nutrition*, 151(9), 2852.
    Lamers, Y., Prinz-Langenohl, R., Brämswig, S., & Pietrzik, K. (2006). Red blood cell folate concentrations increase more after supplementation with [6 S]-5-methyltetrahydrofolate than with folic acid in women of childbearing age. *The American Journal of Clinical Nutrition*, 84(1), 156-161.
3   Valera-Gran, D., Navarrete-Muñoz, E. M., Garcia de la Hera, M., Fernández-Somoano, A., Tardón, A., Ibarluzea, J., ... & Julvez, J. (2017). Effect of maternal high dosages of folic acid supplements on neurocognitive development in children at 4–5 y of age: the prospective birth cohort Infancia y Medio Ambiente (INMA) study. *The American Journal of Clinical Nutrition*, 106(3), 878–887.
4   Bentley, S., Hermes, A., Phillips, D., Daoud, Y. A., & Hanna, S. (2011). Comparative effectiveness of a prenatal medical food to prenatal vitamins on hemoglobin levels and adverse outcomes: a retrospective analysis. *Clinical Therapeutics, 33*(2), 204–210.
5   Ma, G., Chen, Y., Liu, X., Gao, Y., Deavila, J. M., Zhu, M. J., & Du, M. (2022). Vitamin A supplementation during pregnancy in shaping child growth outcomes: A meta-analysis. *Critical Reviews in Food Science and Nutrition*, 1-16.
6   McCauley, M. E., van den Broek, N., Dou, L., & Othman, M. (2015). Vitamin A supplementation during pregnancy for maternal

and newborn outcomes. *Cochrane Database of Systematic Reviews*, (10).

7   Choobdar, F. A., Ghassemzadeh, M., Aslanbeigi, F., Attarian, M., Robatmeili, L., Rahimian, H., … & Anari, A. M. (2022). Association of lower vitamin a levels in neonates and their mothers with increased risk of neonatal late-onset sepsis: A case-control study. *Journal of Mother and Child*, 26(1), 78-86.

8   Rothman, K. J., Moore, L. L., Singer, M. R., Nguyen, U. S. D., Mannino, S., & Milunsky, A. (1995). Teratogenicity of high vitamin A intake. *New England Journal of Medicine*, 333(21), 1369-1373.

9   Ma, G., Chen, Y., Liu, X., Gao, Y., Deavila, J. M., Zhu, M. J., & Du, M. (2022). Vitamin A supplementation during pregnancy in shaping child growth outcomes: A meta-analysis. *Critical Reviews in Food Science and Nutrition*, 1-16.

10 Mayne, S. T., Cartmel, B., Silva, F., Kim, C. S., Fallon, B. G., Briskin, K., … & Goodwin Jr, W. J. (1998). Effect of supplemental β-carotene on plasma concentrations of carotenoids, retinol, and α-tocopherol in humans. *The American Journal of Clinical Nutrition*, 68(3), 642-647.

11 Bastos Maia, S., Rolland Souza, A. S., Costa Caminha, M. D. F., Lins da Silva, S., Callou Cruz, R. D. S. B. L., Carvalho dos Santos, C., & Batista Filho, M. (2019). Vitamin A and pregnancy: a narrative review. *Nutrients*, 11(3), 681.

12 Liu, J., Zhan, S., Jia, Y., Li, Y., Liu, Y., Dong, Y., … & Cao, Z. (2020). Retinol and α-tocopherol in pregnancy: Establishment of reference intervals and associations with CBC. *Maternal & Child Nutrition*, 16(3), e12975.

13 Shaw, G. M., Carmichael, S. L., Yang, W., Selvin, S., & Schaffer, D. M. (2004). Periconceptional dietary intake of choline and betaine and neural tube defects in offspring. *American Journal of Epidemiology, 160*(2), 102-109.

14 Zeisel, S. H. (2006). Choline: critical role during fetal development and dietary requirements in adults. *Annu. Rev. Nutr.*, 26, 229–250. Moreno, H. C., de Brugada, I., Carias, D., & Gallo, M. (2013). Long-lasting effects of prenatal dietary choline availability on object recognition memory ability in adult rats. *Nutritional Neuroscience*, 16(6), 269–274.

Meck, W. H., & Williams, C. L. (1997). Characterization of the facilitative effects of perinatal choline supplementation on timing and temporal memory. *Neuroreport,* 8(13), 2831–2835.

Meck, W. H., & Williams, C. L. (1997). Perinatal choline supplementation increases the threshold for chunking in spatial memory. *Neuroreport,* 8(14), 3053–3059.

Meck, W. H., & Williams, C. L. (1997). Simultaneous temporal processing is sensitive to prenatal choline availability in mature and aged rats. *Neuroreport,* 8(14), 3045–3051.

Meck, W. H., Smith, R. A., & Williams, C. L. (1988). Pre- and postnatal choline supplementation produces long-term facilitation of spatial memory. Developmental Psychobiology: *The Journal of the International Society for Developmental Psychobiology,* 21(4), 339–353.

Zeisel, S. H. (2006). Choline: critical role during fetal development and dietary requirements in adults. *Annu. Rev. Nutr.,* 26, 229–250.

Williams, C. L., Meck, W. H., Heyer, D. D., & Loy, R. (1998). Hypertrophy of basal forebrain neurons and enhanced visuospatial memory in perinatally choline-supplemented rats. *Brain Research,* 794(2), 225–238.

15 Boeke, C. E., Gillman, M. W., Hughes, M. D., Rifas-Shiman, S. L., Villamor, E., & Oken, E. (2012). Choline intake during pregnancy and child cognition at age 7 years. *American Journal of Epidemiology,* 177(12), 1338–1347.

16 Brunst, K. J., Wright, R. O., DiGioia, K., Enlow, M. B., Fernandez, H., Wright, R. J., & Kannan, S. (2014). Racial/ethnic and sociodemographic factors associated with micronutrient intakes and inadequacies among pregnant women in an urban US population. *Public Health Nutrition,* 17(9), 1960–1970.

Wallace, T. C., & Fulgoni, V. L. (2017). Usual choline intakes are associated with egg and protein food consumption in the United States. *Nutrients,* 9(8), 839.

Roeren, M., Kordowski, A., Sina, C., & Smollich, M. (2022). Inadequate Choline Intake in Pregnant Women in Germany. *Nutrients,* 14(22), 4862.

17 Bahnfleth, C. L., Strupp, B. J., Caudill, M. A., & Canfield, R. L. (2022). Prenatal choline supplementation improves child sustained attention: A 7-year follow-up of a randomized controlled feeding trial. *The FASEB Journal,* 36(1).

18 Bahnfleth, C. L., Strupp, B. J., Caudill, M. A., & Canfield, R. L. (2022). Prenatal choline supplementation improves child sustained attention: A 7-year follow-up of a randomized controlled feeding trial. *The FASEB Journal*, 36(1).

19 Smolders, L., de Wit, N. J., Balvers, M. G., Obeid, R., Vissers, M. M., & Esser, D. (2019). Natural choline from egg yolk phospholipids is more efficiently absorbed compared with choline bitartrate; outcomes of a randomized trial in healthy adults. *Nutrients*, 11(11), 2758.

20 Böckmann, K. A., Franz, A. R., Minarski, M., Shunova, A., Maiwald, C. A., Schwarz, J., ... & Bernhard, W. (2022). Differential metabolism of choline supplements in adult volunteers. *European Journal of Nutrition*, 1-12.
    Wilcox, J., Skye, S. M., Graham, B., Zabell, A., Li, X. S., Li, L., ... & Tang, W. W. (2021). Dietary choline supplements, but not eggs, raise fasting TMAO levels in participants with normal renal function: a randomized clinical trial. *The American Journal of Medicine*, 134(9), 1160-1169.
    Tang, W. W., Wang, Z., Levison, B. S., Koeth, R. A., Britt, E. B., Fu, X., ... & Hazen, S. L. (2013). Intestinal microbial metabolism of phosphatidylcholine and cardiovascular risk. *New England Journal of Medicine*, 368(17), 1575-1584.

21 Jääskeläinen, T., Kärkkäinen, O., Heinonen, S., Hanhineva, K., & Laivuori, H. (2022). No association in maternal serum levels of TMAO and its precursors in pre-eclampsia and in non-complicated pregnancies. *Pregnancy Hypertension*, 28, 74-80.

22 Lemos, B. S., Medina-Vera, I., Malysheva, O. V., Caudill, M. A., & Fernandez, M. L. (2018). Effects of egg consumption and choline supplementation on plasma choline and trimethylamine-N-oxide in a young population. *Journal of the American College of Nutrition*, 37(8), 716-723.

Chapter 2. Preventing Preterm Birth with Omega-3s

1 Olsen, S., Sorensen, T. A., Secher, N., Hansen, H., Jensen, B., Sommer, S., & Knudsen, L. (1986). Intake of marine fat, rich in (n-3)-polyunsaturated fatty acids, may increase birthweight by prolonging gestation. *The Lancet*, 328(8503), 367–369.

2 Middleton, P. Gomersall JC, Gould JF, Shepherd E, Olsen SF, Makrides M. (2018) Omega-3 fatty acid addition during pregnancy. *Cochrane Database Syst Rev. 2018* Nov 15.

Carlson, S. E., Gajewski, B. J., Valentine, C. J., Sands, S. A., Brown, A. R., Kerling, E. H., ... & Rogers, L. K. (2023). Early and late preterm birth rates in participants adherent to randomly assigned high dose docosahexaenoic acid (DHA) supplementation in pregnancy. *Clinical Nutrition*, 42(2), 235-243.

Simmonds, L. A., Sullivan, T. R., Skubisz, M., Middleton, P. F., Best, K. P., Yelland, L. N., ... & Makrides, M. (2020). Omega-3 fatty acid supplementation in pregnancy—baseline omega-3 status and early preterm birth: exploratory analysis of a randomised controlled trial. *BJOG: An International Journal of Obstetrics & Gynaecology*, 127(8), 975-981.

3   Olsen, S. F., Halldorsson, T. I., Thorne-Lyman, A. L., Strøm, M., Gørtz, S., Granstrøm, C., ... & Cohen, A. S. (2018). Plasma Concentrations of Long Chain N-3 Fatty Acids in Early and Mid-Pregnancy and Risk of Early Preterm Birth. *EBioMedicine*, 35, 325–333.

4   https://www.cochrane.org/news/new-research-finds-omega-3-fatty-acids-reduce-risk-premature-birth

5   Lauterbach, R. (2018). EPA+ DHA in Prevention of Early Preterm Birth–Do We Know How to Apply it? *EBioMedicine*, 35, 16–17.

6   Judge, M. P., Harel, O., & Lammi-Keefe, C. J. (2007). Maternal consumption of a docosahexaenoic acid–containing functional food during pregnancy: benefit for infant performance on problem-solving but not on recognition memory tasks at age 9 mo. *The American Journal of Clinical Nutrition*, 85(6), 1572–1577.

Hibbeln, J. R., Davis, J. M., Steer, C., Emmett, P., Rogers, I., Williams, C., & Golding, J. (2007). Maternal seafood consumption in pregnancy and neurodevelopmental outcomes in childhood (ALSPAC study): an observational cohort study. *The Lancet*, 369(9561), 578–585.

Dunstan, J. A., Simmer, K., Dixon, G., & Prescott, S. L. (2008). Cognitive assessment of children at age 2½ years after maternal fish oil supplementation in pregnancy: a randomised controlled trial. *Archives of Disease in Childhood-Fetal and Neonatal Edition*, 93(1), F45–F50.

7   Helland, I. B., Smith, L., Saarem, K., Saugstad, O. D., & Drevon, C. A. (2003). Maternal supplementation with very-long-chain n-3 fatty acids during pregnancy and lactation augments children's IQ at 4 years of age. *PEDIATRICS-SPRINGFIELD*, 111(1), 189–189.

8   Klemens, C. M., Berman, D. R., & Mozurkewich, E. L. (2011).
    The effect of perinatal omega-3 fatty acid supplementation on
    inflammatory markers and allergic diseases: a systematic review.
    BJOG: An International Journal of Obstetrics & Gynaecology,
    118(8), 916-925.
    Huynh, L. B. P., Nguyen, N. N., Fan, H. Y., Huang, S. Y., Huang,
    C. H., & Chen, Y. C. (2023). Maternal omega-3 supplementation
    during pregnancy, but not childhood supplementation, reduces the
    risk of food allergy diseases in offspring. *The Journal of Allergy
    and Clinical Immunology: In Practice*, 11(9), 2862-2871.

9   Gao, L.; Lin, L.; Shan, N.; Ren, C.-Y.; Long, X.; Sun, Y.-H.; Wang,
    L. The impact of omega-3 fatty acid supplementation on glycemic
    control in patients with gestational diabetes: A systematic review
    and meta-analysis of randomized controlled studies. *J. Matern.
    Neonatal Med.* 2018, 33, 1767–1773.

10 Jamilian, M., Samimi, M., Kolahdooz, F., Khalaji, F., Razavi, M.,
    & Asemi, Z. (2016). Omega-3 fatty acid supplementation affects
    pregnancy outcomes in gestational diabetes: a randomized,
    double-blind, placebo-controlled trial. *The Journal of Maternal-
    Fetal & Neonatal Medicine*, 29(4), 669-675.

11 Carlson, S. E., Gajewski, B. J., Valentine, C. J., Sands, S. A., Brown,
    A. R., Kerling, E. H., ... & Rogers, L. K. (2023). Early and late
    preterm birth rates in participants adherent to randomly assigned
    high dose docosahexaenoic acid (DHA) supplementation in
    pregnancy. *Clinical Nutrition*, 42(2), 235-243.
    Carlson, S. E., Colombo, J., Gajewski, B. J., Gustafson, K.
    M., Mundy, D., Yeast, J., ... & Shaddy, D. J. (2013). DHA
    supplementation and pregnancy outcomes. *The American Journal
    of Clinical Nutrition*, 97(4), 808–815.

12 Middleton, P., Gomersall, J. C., Gould, J. F., Shepherd, E., Olsen,
    S. F., & Makrides, M. (2018). Omega-3 fatty acid addition during
    pregnancy. *Cochrane Database of Systematic Reviews*, (11).

13 De Groot, R. H., Hornstra, G., van Houwelingen, A. C., &
    Roumen, F. (2004). Effect of α-linolenic acid supplementation
    during pregnancy on maternal and neonatal polyunsaturated fatty
    acid status and pregnancy outcome. *The American Journal of
    Clinical Nutrition*, 79(2), 251–260.

14 Bays, H. E. (2007). Safety considerations with omega-3 fatty acid
    therapy. *The American Journal of Cardiology*, 99(6), S35–S43.

15 Olsen, S. F., Secher, N. J., Tabor, A., Weber, T., Walker, J. J., & Gluud, C. (2000). Randomised clinical trials of fish oil supplementation in high risk pregnancies. *BJOG: An International Journal of Obstetrics & Gynaecology,* 107(3), 382–395.

16 Middleton, P., Gomersall, J. C., Gould, J. F., Shepherd, E., Olsen, S. F., & Makrides, M. (2019). Omega-3 fatty acid addition during pregnancy. *Obstetrical & Gynecological Survey,* 74(4), 189-191.

17 Huynh, L. B. P., Nguyen, N. N., Fan, H. Y., Huang, S. Y., Huang, C. H., & Chen, Y. C. (2023). Maternal omega-3 supplementation during pregnancy, but not childhood supplementation, reduces the risk of food allergy diseases in offspring. *The Journal of Allergy and Clinical Immunology: In Practice,* 11(9), 2862-2871.

18 https://www.epa.gov/international-cooperation/mercury-emissions-global-context

19 FDA (2014). *New Advice: Pregnant Women and Young Children Should Eat More Fish.* https://www.fda.gov/consumers/consumer-updates/new-advice-pregnant-women-and-young-children-should-eat-more-fish

20 Harauma, A., Yoshihara, H., Hoshi, Y., Hamazaki, K., & Moriguchi, T. (2023). Effects of Varied Omega-3 Fatty Acid Supplementation on Postpartum Mental Health and the Association between Prenatal Erythrocyte Omega-3 Fatty Acid Levels and Postpartum Mental Health. *Nutrients,* 15(20), 4388.
Vaz, J. D. S., Farias, D. R., Adegboye, A. R. A., Nardi, A. E., & Kac, G. (2017). Omega-3 supplementation from pregnancy to postpartum to prevent depressive symptoms: a randomized placebo-controlled trial. *BMC Pregnancy and Childbirth,* 17(1), 1-13.
Sousa, T. M. D., & Santos, L. C. D. (2023). Effect of antenatal omega-3 supplementation on maternal depressive symptoms from pregnancy to 6 months postpartum: a randomized double-blind placebo-controlled trial. Nutritional *Neuroscience,* 26(6), 551-559.

21 Harauma, A., Yoshihara, H., Hoshi, Y., Hamazaki, K., & Moriguchi, T. (2023). Effects of Varied Omega-3 Fatty Acid Supplementation on Postpartum Mental Health and the Association between Prenatal Erythrocyte Omega-3 Fatty Acid Levels and Postpartum Mental Health. *Nutrients,* 15(20), 4388.

Chapter 3. Choosing the Best Prenatal Supplement

1 Bodnar, L. M., & Simhan, H. N. (2010). Vitamin D may be a link to black-white disparities in adverse birth outcomes. *Obstetrical & Gynecological Survey*, 65(4), 273-284.

2 Bodnar, L. M., Simhan, H. N., Powers, R. W., Frank, M. P., Cooperstein, E., & Roberts, J. M. (2007). High prevalence of vitamin D insufficiency in black and white pregnant women residing in the northern United States and their neonates. *The Journal of Nutrition*, 137(2), 447–452.

3 Wagner, C. L., Baggerly, C., McDonnell, S. L., Baggerly, L., Hamilton, S. A., Winkler, J., ... & Hollis, B. W. (2015). Post-hoc comparison of vitamin D status at three timepoints during pregnancy demonstrates lower risk of preterm birth with higher vitamin D closer to delivery. *The Journal of steroid biochemistry and molecular biology*, 148, 256-260.

4 McDonnell, S. L., Baggerly, K. A., Baggerly, C. A., Aliano, J. L., French, C. B., Baggerly, L. L., ... & Wineland, R. J. (2017). Maternal 25 (OH) D concentrations≥ 40 ng/mL associated with 60% lower preterm birth risk among general obstetrical patients at an urban medical center. *PloS One*, 12(7), e0180483.

5 McDonnell, S. L., Baggerly, K. A., Baggerly, C. A., Aliano, J. L., French, C. B., Baggerly, L. L., ... & Wineland, R. J. (2017). Maternal 25 (OH) D concentrations≥ 40 ng/mL associated with 60% lower preterm birth risk among general obstetrical patients at an urban medical center. *PloS One*, 12(7), e0180483.

6 Sorokin, Y., Romero, R., Mele, L., Wapner, R. J., Iams, J. D., Dudley, D. J., ... & Caritis, S. N. (2010). Maternal serum interleukin-6, C-reactive protein, and matrix metalloproteinase-9 concentrations as risk factors for preterm birth< 32 weeks and adverse neonatal outcomes. *American Journal of Perinatology*, 27(08), 631–640. Lee, H. J., Han, J. Y., Hwang, J. H., Kwon, H. Y., & Choi, H. Z. (2022). Association between Preterm Premature Rupture of Membranes and Vitamin D Levels in Maternal Plasma and Umbilical Cord Blood of Newborns: A Prospective Study. *Clinical and Experimental Obstetrics & Gynecology*, 49(7), 158

7 Bodnar, L. M., Platt, R. W., & Simhan, H. N. (2015). Early-pregnancy vitamin D deficiency and risk of preterm birth subtypes. *Obstetrics and Gynecology*, 125(2), 439.

Qin, L. L., Lu, F. G., Yang, S. H., Xu, H. L., & Luo, B. A. (2016). Does maternal vitamin D deficiency increase the risk of preterm birth: a meta-analysis of observational studies. *Nutrients, 8*(5), 301.

8 Woo, J., Giurgescu, C., & Wagner, C. L. (2019). Evidence of an association between vitamin D deficiency and preterm birth and preeclampsia: a critical review. *Journal of Midwifery & Women's Health*, 64(5), 613-629.

9 Litonjua, A. A., Carey, V. J., Laranjo, N., Harshfield, B. J., McElrath, T. F., O'Connor, G. T., ... & Weiss, S. T. (2016). Effect of prenatal supplementation with vitamin D on asthma or recurrent wheezing in offspring by age 3 years: the VDAART randomized clinical trial. *Jama*, 315(4), 362-370.

10 Wang, S., Xin, X., Luo, W., Mo, M., Si, S., Shao, B., ... & Yu, Y. (2021). Association of vitamin D and gene variants in the vitamin D metabolic pathway with preterm birth. *Nutrition*, 89, 111349.

11 Holick, M. F., Binkley, N. C., Bischoff-Ferrari, H. A., Gordon, C. M., Hanley, D. A., Heaney, R. P., ... & Weaver, C. M. (2011). Evaluation, treatment, and prevention of vitamin D deficiency: an Endocrine Society clinical practice guideline. *The Journal of Clinical Endocrinology & Metabolism, 96*(7), 1911–1930.

12 Garland, C. F., French, C. B., Baggerly, L. L., & Heaney, R. P. (2011). Vitamin D supplement doses and serum 25-hydroxyvitamin D in the range associated with cancer prevention. *Anticancer Research, 31*(2), 607–611.

13 Tripkovic, L., Lambert, H., Hart, K., Smith, C. P., Bucca, G., Penson, S., ... & Lanham-New, S. (2012). Comparison of vitamin D2 and vitamin D3 supplementation in raising serum 25-hydroxyvitamin D status: a systematic review and meta-analysis. *The American Journal of Clinical Nutrition, 95*(6), 1357–1364. Chapter 4. Baby Brain Food: Fish & Omega-3 Fats

14 Wang, M., Chen, Z., Hu, Y., Wang, Y., Wu, Y., Lian, F., ... & Xu, X. (2021). The effects of vitamin D supplementation on glycemic control and maternal-neonatal outcomes in women with established gestational diabetes mellitus: A systematic review and meta-analysis. *Clinical Nutrition*, 40(5), 3148-3157.
Wang, L., Zhang, C., Song, Y., & Zhang, Z. (2020). Serum vitamin D deficiency and risk of gestational diabetes mellitus: a meta-analysis. *Archives of Medical Science*, 16(1).

Rodrigues, C. Z., Cardoso, M. A., Maruyama, J. M., Neves, P. A., Qi, L., & Lourenço, B. H. (2022). Vitamin D insufficiency, excessive weight gain, and insulin resistance during pregnancy. *Nutrition, Metabolism and Cardiovascular Diseases*, 32(9), 2121-2128.

Dahma, G., Neamtu, R., Nitu, R., Gluhovschi, A., Bratosin, F., Grigoras, M. L., … & Bernad, E. (2022). The influence of maternal vitamin D supplementation in pregnancies associated with preeclampsia: A case-control study. *Nutrients*, 14(15), 3008.

Merewood, A., Mehta, S. D., Chen, T. C., Bauchner, H., & Holick, M. F. (2009). Association between vitamin D deficiency and primary cesarean section. *The Journal of Clinical Endocrinology & Metabolism*, 94(3), 940-945.

15 Wang, M., Chen, Z., Hu, Y., Wang, Y., Wu, Y., Lian, F., … & Xu, X. (2021). The effects of vitamin D supplementation on glycemic control and maternal-neonatal outcomes in women with established gestational diabetes mellitus: A systematic review and meta-analysis. *Clinical Nutrition*, 40(5), 3148-3157.

16 Belderbos, M.E.; Houben, M.L.; Wilbrink, B.; Lentjes, E.; Bloemen, E.M.; Kimpen, J.L.L.; Rovers, M.; Bont, L. Cord blood Vitamin D deficiency is associated with respiratory syncytial virus bronchiolitis. *Pediatrics* 2011, 127, 1513–1520.

Mansur, J. L., Oliveri, B., Giacoia, E., Fusaro, D., & Costanzo, P. R. (2022). Vitamin D: before, during and after pregnancy: effect on neonates and children. *Nutrients*, 14(9), 1900.

17 Willemse, J. P., Meertens, L. J., Scheepers, H. C., Achten, N. M., Eussen, S. J., van Dongen, M. C., & Smits, L. J. (2020). Calcium intake from diet and supplement use during early pregnancy: The Expect study I. *European Journal of Nutrition*, 59, 167-174.

18 Dwarkanath, P., Muhihi, A., Sudfeld, C. R., Wylie, B. J., Wang, M., Perumal, N., … & Fawzi, W. W. (2024). Two Randomized Trials of Low-Dose Calcium Supplementation in Pregnancy. *New England Journal of Medicine*, 390(2), 143-153.

19 Woo Kinshella, M. L., Sarr, C., Sandhu, A., Bone, J. N., Vidler, M., Moore, S. E., … & PRECISE Network. (2022). Calcium for pre-eclampsia prevention: a systematic review and network meta-analysis to guide personalised antenatal care. *BJOG: An International Journal of Obstetrics & Gynaecology*, 129(11), 1833-1843.

Hofmeyr, G. J., Betrán, A. P., Singata-Madliki, M., Cormick, G., Munjanja, S. P., Fawcus, S., … & Tahuringana, E. (2019).

Prepregnancy and early pregnancy calcium supplementation among women at high risk of pre-eclampsia: a multicentre, double-blind, randomised, placebo-controlled trial. *The Lancet*, 393(10169), 330-339.

20 Dwarkanath, P., Muhihi, A., Sudfeld, C. R., Wylie, B. J., Wang, M., Perumal, N., ... & Fawzi, W. W. (2024). Two Randomized Trials of Low-Dose Calcium Supplementation in Pregnancy. *New England Journal of Medicine*, 390(2), 143-153.

21 Mazza, G. R., Solorio, C., Stek, A. M., Kalayjian, L. A., Wilson, M. L., & Gordon, B. J. (2023). Assessing the efficacy of magnesium oxide and riboflavin as preventative treatment of migraines in pregnancy. *Archives of Gynecology and Obstetrics*, 308(6), 1749-1754.

Chapter 4. Aspirin, Preeclampsia, and Placenta Health

1 Shih, T., Peneva, D., Xu, X., Sutton, A., Triche, E., Ehrenkranz, R. A., ... & Stevens, W. (2015). The rising burden of preeclampsia in the United States impacts both maternal and child health. *American Journal of Perinatology*, 329-338.

2 Reddy, M., Wright, L., Rolnik, D. L., Li, W., Mol, B. W., La Gerche, A., ... & Palmer, K. (2019). Evaluation of cardiac function in women with a history of preeclampsia: a systematic review and meta-analysis. *Journal of the American Heart Association*, 8(22), e013545.

3 Aksu, E., Cuglan, B., Tok, A., Celik, E., Doganer, A., Sokmen, A., & Sokmen, G. (2022). Cardiac electrical and structural alterations in preeclampsia. *The Journal of Maternal-Fetal & Neonatal Medicine*, 35(1), 1-10.
deMartelly, V. A., Dreixler, J., Tung, A., Mueller, A., Heimberger, S., Fazal, A. A., ... & Shahul, S. (2021). Long-term postpartum cardiac function and its association with preeclampsia. *Journal of the American Heart Association*, 10(5), e018526.

4 Giorgione, V., Ridder, A., Kalafat, E., Khalil, A., & Thilaganathan, B. (2021). Incidence of postpartum hypertension within 2 years of a pregnancy complicated by pre-eclampsia: a systematic review and meta-analysis. *BJOG: An International Journal of Obstetrics & Gynaecology*, 128(3), 495-503.

5 Duckitt, K., & Harrington, D. (2005). Risk factors for pre-eclampsia at antenatal booking: systematic review of controlled studies. *BMJ*, 330(7491), 565.

6   Watanabe, N., Fujiwara, T., Suzuki, T., Jwa, S. C., Taniguchi,
     K., Yamanobe, Y., … & Sago, H. (2014). Is in vitro fertilization
     associated with preeclampsia? A propensity score matched study.
     BMC Pregnancy and Childbirth, 14, 1-7.
7   Woods, L., Perez-Garcia, V., Kieckbusch, J., Wang, X., DeMayo,
     F., Colucci, F., & Hemberger, M. (2017). Decidualisation and
     placentation defects are a major cause of age-related reproductive
     decline. *Nature Communications*, 8(1), 352.
     Staff, A. C., Fjeldstad, H. E., Fosheim, I. K., Moe, K., Turowski, G.,
     Johnsen, G. M., … & Sugulle, M. (2022). Failure of physiological
     transformation and spiral artery atherosis: their roles in
     preeclampsia. *American Journal of Obstetrics and Gynecology*,
     226(2), S895-S906.
     Cooke, C. L. M., & Davidge, S. T. (2019). Advanced maternal
     age and the impact on maternal and offspring cardiovascular
     health. American Journal of Physiology-Heart and Circulatory
     Physiology, 317(2), H387-H394.
8   Rana, S., Lemoine, E., Granger, J. P., & Karumanchi, S. A. (2019).
     Preeclampsia: pathophysiology, challenges, and perspectives.
     Circulation Research, 124(7), 1094-1112.
9   Keukens, A., Va. Wely, M., Va. de. Meulen, C., & Mochtar, M. H.
     (2021). P–762 Preeclampsia in pregnancies resulting from oocyte
     donation, IVF or natural conception. A systematic review and meta-
     analysis. *Human Reproduction*, 36(Supplement_1), deab130-761.
10   Gunnarsdottir, J., Stephansson, O., Cnattingius, S., Åkerud, H., &
     Wikström, A. K. (2014). Risk of placental dysfunction disorders
     after prior miscarriages: a population-based study. *American
     Journal of Obstetrics and Gynecology*, 211(1), 34-e1.
     Schramm, A. M., & Clowse, M. E. (2014). Aspirin for prevention
     of preeclampsia in lupus pregnancy. *Autoimmune Diseases*, 2014.
     Spradley, F. T., Palei, A. C., & Granger, J. P. (2015). Immune
     mechanisms linking obesity and preeclampsia. *Biomolecules*, 5(4),
     3142-3176.
11   Yuan, J., Yu, Y., Zhu, T., Lin, X., Jing, X., & Zhang, J. (2022). Oral
     magnesium supplementation for the prevention of preeclampsia:
     a meta-analysis or randomized controlled trials. *Biological Trace
     Element Research*, 200(8), 3572-3581.
12   Rolnik, D. L., Wright, D., Poon, L. C., O'Gorman, N., Syngelaki,
     A., de Paco Matallana, C., … & Nicolaides, K. H. (2017).

Aspirin versus placebo in pregnancies at high risk for preterm preeclampsia. *New England Journal of Medicine*, 377(7), 613-622.

13 Wheeler, S. M., Myers, S. O., Swamy, G. K., & Myers, E. R. (2022). Estimated prevalence of risk factors for preeclampsia among individuals giving birth in the US in 2019. *JAMA Network Open*, 5(1), e2142343-e2142343.

14 Keukens, A., Van Wely, M., Van Der Meulen, C., & Mochtar, M. H. (2022). Pre-eclampsia in pregnancies resulting from oocyte donation, natural conception or IVF: a systematic review and meta-analysis. *Human Reproduction*, 37(3), 586-599.

Chih, H. J., Elias, F., Gaudet, L., & Velez, M. (2021). Risk of preeclampsia in pregnancies conceived by assisted reproductive technology: a systematic review and meta-analysis of cohort studies. *Journal of Obstetrics and Gynaecology Canada*, 43(5), 653.

Singh, B., Reschke, L., Segars, J., & Baker, V. L. (2020). Frozen-thawed embryo transfer: the potential importance of the corpus luteum in preventing obstetrical complications. *Fertility and Sterility*, 113(2), 252-257.

Mills, G., Badeghiesh, A., Suarthana, E., Baghlaf, H., & Dahan, M. H. (2020). Polycystic ovary syndrome as an independent risk factor for gestational diabetes and hypertensive disorders of pregnancy: a population-based study on 9.1 million pregnancies. *Human Reproduction*, 35(7), 1666-1674.

15 Rolnik, D. L., Wright, D., Poon, L. C., O'Gorman, N., Syngelaki, A., de Paco Matallana, C., … & Nicolaides, K. H. (2017). Aspirin versus placebo in pregnancies at high risk for preterm preeclampsia. *New England Journal of Medicine*, 377(7), 613-622.

16 Roberge S, Nicolaides K, Demers S, Hyett J, Chaillet N, Bujold E. The role of aspirin dose on the prevention of preeclampsia and fetal growth restriction: systematic review and meta-analysis. *Am J Obstet* Gynecol 2017; 216: 110– 20.e6.

Duley, L., Meher, S., Hunter, K. E., Seidler, A. L., & Askie, L. M. (2019). Antiplatelet agents for preventing pre-eclampsia and its complications. *Cochrane Database of Systematic Reviews*, (10).

Hoffman MK, Goudar SS, Kodkany BS. , et al; ASPIRIN Study Group. Low-dose aspirin for the prevention of preterm delivery in nulliparous women with a singleton pregnancy (ASPIRIN): a randomised, double-blind, placebo-controlled trial. *Lancet* 2020; 395 (10220): 285-293

17 He, H., Qi, D., Fang, M., Tian, Y., Yan, L., Ma, J., & Du, Y. (2023). The
    Effect of Short-Term Aspirin Administration during Programmed
    Frozen-Thawed Embryo Transfer on Pregnancy Outcomes and
    Complications. *Journal of Clinical Medicine*, 12(3), 1064.
    Davar, R., Pourmasumi, S., Mohammadi, B., & Lahijani, M. M.
    (2020). The effect of low-dose aspirin on the pregnancy rate in
    frozen-thawed embryo transfer cycles: A randomized clinical trial.
    International Journal of Reproductive Biomedicine, 18(9), 693.
    Madani, T., Ahmadi, F., Jahangiri, N., Bahmanabadi, A., &
    Bagheri Lankarani, N. (2019). Does low-dose aspirin improve
    pregnancy rate in women undergoing frozen-thawed embryo
    transfer cycle? A pilot double-blind, randomized placebo-
    controlled trial. *Journal of Obstetrics and Gynaecology Research*,
    45(1), 156-163.
    Kim, M. J., Lee, H. J., Yu, Y., Seo, B. K., Cha, S. H., Kim, H. S., ...
    & Yang, K. M. (2005). Effect of Low-dose Aspirin on Implantation
    and Pregnancy Rates in Patients Undergoing Frozen-thawed
    Embryo Transfer. *Korean Journal of Fertility and Sterility*, 32(3),
    243-252.
    Schisterman, E. F., Silver, R. M., Lesher, L. L., Faraggi, D.,
    Wactawski-Wende, J., Townsend, J. M., ... & Galai, N. (2014).
    Preconception low-dose aspirin and pregnancy outcomes: results
    from the EAGeR randomised trial. The Lancet, 384(9937), 29-36.
18 Truong, A., Sayago, M. M., Kutteh, W. H., & Ke, R. W. (2016).
    Subchorionic hematomas are increased in early pregnancy in
    women taking low-dose aspirin. *Fertility and Sterility*, 105(5),
    1241-1246.
19 E. Rhodes, C. Kasales, M.B. Porter, S. Kupesic, R.D. Harris, First-
    Trimester Sonographic Finding Associated with Poor Intrauterine
    Outcome, *Radiologist*, 9 (2002), pp. 309-315
20 Truong, A., Sayago, M. M., Kutteh, W. H., & Ke, R. W. (2016).
    Subchorionic hematomas are increased in early pregnancy in
    women taking low-dose aspirin. *Fertility and Sterility*, 105(5),
    1241-1246.
21 Zhou, J., Wu, M., Wang, B., Hou, X., Wang, J., Chen, H., ... &
    Sun, H. (2017). The effect of first trimester subchorionic hematoma
    on pregnancy outcomes in patients underwent IVF/ICSI
    treatment. *The Journal of Maternal-Fetal & Neonatal Medicine*,
    30(4), 406-410.

Fu, Z., Ding, X., Wei, D., Li, J., Cang, R., & Li, X. (2023). Impact of subchorionic hematoma on pregnancy outcomes in women with recurrent pregnancy loss. *Biomolecules and Biomedicine*, 23(1), 170.

22 Heller, H. T., Asch, E. A., Durfee, S. M., Goldenson, R. P., Peters, H. E., Ginsburg, E. S., ... & Benson, C. B. (2018). Subchorionic hematoma: correlation of grading techniques with first-trimester pregnancy outcome. *Journal of Ultrasound in Medicine*, 37(7), 1725-1732.

23 Fu, Z., Ding, X., Wei, D., Li, J., Cang, R., & Li, X. (2023). Impact of subchorionic hematoma on pregnancy outcomes in women with recurrent pregnancy loss. *Biomolecules and Biomedicine*, 23(1), 170. Inman, E. R., Miranian, D. C., Stevenson, M. J., Kobernik, E. K., Moravek, M. B., & Schon, S. B. (2022). Outcomes of subchorionic hematoma-affected pregnancies in the infertile population. *International Journal of Gynecology & Obstetrics*, 159(3), 743-750. Anderson, K. L., Jimenez, P. T., Omurtag, K. R., & Jungheim, E. S. (2020). Outcomes of in vitro fertilization pregnancies complicated by subchorionic hematoma detected on first-trimester ultrasound. *F&S Reports*, 1(2), 149-153.

24 Tulppala, M., Marttunen, M., Söderstrom-Anttila, V., Foudila, T., Ailus, K., Palosuo, T., & Ylikorkala, O. (1997). Low-dose aspirin in prevention of miscarriage in women with unexplained or autoimmune related recurrent miscarriage: effect on prostacyclin and thromboxane A2 production. Human reproduction (Oxford, England), 12(7), 1567-1572. Schisterman, E. F., Silver, R. M., Lesher, L. L., Faraggi, D., Wactawski-Wende, J., Townsend, J. M., ... & Galai, N. (2014). Preconception low-dose aspirin and pregnancy outcomes: results from the EAGeR randomised trial. The Lancet, 384(9937), 29-36

25 Truong, A., Sayago, M. M., Kutteh, W. H., & Ke, R. W. (2016). Subchorionic hematomas are increased in early pregnancy in women taking low-dose aspirin. *Fertility and Sterility*, 105(5), 1241-1246. Rai, R., Cohen, H., Dave, M., & Regan, L. (1997). Randomised controlled trial of aspirin and aspirin plus heparin in pregnant women with recurrent miscarriage associated with phospholipid antibodies (or antiphospholipid antibodies). Bmj, 314(7076), 253.

26 Mendoza, M., Bonacina, E., Garcia-Manau, P., López, M., Caamiña, S., Vives, À., ... & Suy, A. (2023). Aspirin

discontinuation at 24 to 28 weeks' gestation in pregnancies at high risk of preterm preeclampsia: a randomized clinical trial. *JAMA*, 329(7), 542-550.

27 Menichini, D., Feliciello, L., Neri, I., & Facchinetti, F. (2023). L-Arginine supplementation in pregnancy: a systematic review of maternal and fetal outcomes. *The Journal of Maternal-Fetal & Neonatal Medicine*, 36(1), 2217465.

28 Camarena Pulido, E. E., García Benavides, L., Panduro Barón, J. G., Pascoe Gonzalez, S., Madrigal Saray, A. J., García Padilla, F. E., & Totsuka Sutto, S. E. (2016). Efficacy of L-arginine for preventing preeclampsia in high-risk pregnancies: a double-blind, randomized, clinical trial. *Hypertension in Pregnancy*, 35(2), 217-225.

29 Menichini, D., Feliciello, L., Neri, I., & Facchinetti, F. (2023). L-Arginine supplementation in pregnancy: a systematic review of maternal and fetal outcomes. The Journal of Maternal-Fetal & Neonatal Medicine, 36(1), 2217465.
Goto, E. (2021). Effects of prenatal oral l-arginine on birth outcomes: a meta-analysis. *Scientific Reports*, 11(1), 22748.

30 Menichini, D., Feliciello, L., Neri, I., & Facchinetti, F. (2023). L-Arginine supplementation in pregnancy: a systematic review of maternal and fetal outcomes. *The Journal of Maternal-Fetal & Neonatal Medicine*, 36(1), 2217465.

31 Aune, D., Saugstad, O. D., Henriksen, T., & Tonstad, S. (2014). Physical activity and the risk of preeclampsia: a systematic review and meta-analysis. *Epidemiology*, 25(3), 331-343.

32 Yeo, S., Davidge, S., Ronis, D. L., Antonakos, C. L., Hayashi, R., & O'Leary, S. (2008). A comparison of walking versus stretching exercises to reduce the incidence of preeclampsia: a randomized clinical trial. *Hypertension in Pregnancy*, 27(2), 113-130.

33 Hindun, S., & Franciska, Y. (2023). Effect of yoga practice in reducing blood pressure, platelet blood count, and proteinuria in pregnant women with mild preeclampsia. *Journal of Integrative Nursing*, 5(1), 33-36.

34 Karthiga, K., Pal, G. K., Dasari, P., Nanda, N., Velkumary, S., Chinnakali, P., ... & Harichandrakumar, K. T. (2022). Effects of yoga on cardiometabolic risks and fetomaternal outcomes are associated with serum nitric oxide in gestational hypertension: A randomized control trial. *Scientific Reports*, 12(1), 11732.

Chapter 5. Myo-Inositol for Gestational Diabetes

1   Sonagra, A. D., Biradar, S. M., Dattatreya, K., & DS, J. M. (2014). Normal pregnancy-a state of insulin resistance. Journal of clinical and diagnostic research: *JCDR*, 8(11), CC01.

2   Köck, K., Köck, F., Klein, K., Bancher-Todesca, D., & Helmer, H. (2010). Diabetes mellitus and the risk of preterm birth with regard to the risk of spontaneous preterm birth. *The Journal of Maternal-Fetal & Neonatal Medicine*, 23(9), 1004-1008.
    Hedderson, M. M., Ferrara, A., & Sacks, D. A. (2003). Gestational diabetes mellitus and lesser degrees of pregnancy hyperglycemia: association with increased risk of spontaneous preterm birth. *Obstetrics & Gynecology*, 102(4), 850-856.

3   Li, Y., Ren, X., He, L., Li, J., Zhang, S., & Chen, W. (2020). Maternal age and the risk of gestational diabetes mellitus: a systematic review and meta-analysis of over 120 million participants. *Diabetes Research and Clinical Practice*, 162, 108044.

4   Li, Y., Ren, X., He, L., Li, J., Zhang, S., & Chen, W. (2020). Maternal age and the risk of gestational diabetes mellitus: a systematic review and meta-analysis of over 120 million participants. *Diabetes Research and Clinical Practice*, 162, 108044.

5   Unfer, V., Facchinetti, F., Orrù, B., Giordani, B., & Nestler, J. (2017). Myo-inositol effects in women with PCOS: a meta-analysis of randomized controlled trials. *Endocrine Connections*, 6(8), 647-658.

6   D'Anna R, Benedetto V, Rizzo P, Raffone E, Interdonato ML, Corrado F, Di Benedetto A. Myo-inositol may prevent gestational diabetes in PCOS women. *Gynecol Endocrinol* 2012; 28:440–2.

7   D'Anna, R., Scilipoti, A., Giordano, D., Caruso, C., Cannata, M. L., Interdonato, M. L., ... & Di Benedetto, A. (2013). myo-Inositol supplementation and onset of gestational diabetes mellitus in pregnant women with a family history of type 2 diabetes: a prospective, randomized, placebo-controlled study. *Diabetes Care*, 36(4), 854-857.
    Zhang, H., Lv, Y., Li, Z., Sun, L., & Guo, W. (2019). The efficacy of myo-inositol supplementation to prevent gestational diabetes onset: a meta-analysis of randomized controlled trials. *The Journal of Maternal-Fetal & Neonatal Medicine*, 32(13), 2249-2255.

8   Pintaudi, B., Di Vieste, G., Corrado, F., Lucisano, G., Giunta, L., D'ANNA, R., & Di Benedetto, A. (2018). Effects of myo-inositol on

glucose variability in women with gestational diabetes. *European Review for Medical and Pharmacological Sciences*, 22(19), 6567-6572.
Costabile, L., & Unfer, V. (2017). Treatment of gestational diabetes mellitus with myo-inositol: analyzing the cutting edge starting from a peculiar case. *European Review for Medical and Pharmacological Sciences*, 21(Supplement 2), 73-76.
Corrado, F., D'Anna, R., Di Vieste, G., Giordano, D., Pintaudi, B., Santamaria, A., & Di Benedetto, A. (2011). The effect of myoinositol supplementation on insulin resistance in patients with gestational diabetes. *Diabetic Medicine*, 28(8), 972-975.

9   Matarrelli, B., Vitacolonna, E., D'angelo, M., Pavone, G., Mattei, P. A., Liberati, M., & Celentano, C. (2013). Effect of dietary myo-inositol supplementation in pregnancy on the incidence of maternal gestational diabetes mellitus and fetal outcomes: a randomized controlled trial. *The Journal of Maternal-Fetal & Neonatal Medicine*, 26(10), 967-972.
Lubin, V., Shojai, R., Darmon, P., & Cosson, E. (2016). A pilot study of gestational diabetes mellitus not controlled by diet alone: first-line medical treatment with myoinositol may limit the need for insulin. *Diabetes & Metabolism*, 42(3), 192-195.

10 Vitagliano, A., Saccone, G., Cosmi, E., Visentin, S., Dessole, F., Ambrosini, G., & Berghella, V. (2019). Inositol for the prevention of gestational diabetes: a systematic review and meta-analysis of randomized controlled trials. *Archives of Gynecology and Obstetrics*, 299(1), 55-68.

11 Mashayekh-Amiri, S., Delavar, M. A., Bakouei, F., Faramarzi, M., & Esmaeilzadeh, S. (2022). The impact of myo-inositol supplementation on sleep quality in pregnant women: a randomized, double-blind, placebo-controlled study. *The Journal of Maternal-Fetal & Neonatal Medicine*, 35(18), 3415-3423.

12 Esteghamati, A., Aryan, Z., Esteghamati, A. R., & Nakhjavani, M. (2015). Vitamin D deficiency is associated with insulin resistance in nondiabetics and reduced insulin production in type 2 diabetics. *Hormone and Metabolic Research*, 47(04), 273-279.
Marcotorchino, J., Gouranton, E., Romier, B., Tourniaire, F., Astier, J., Malezet, C., ... & Landrier, J. F. (2012). Vitamin D reduces the inflammatory response and restores glucose uptake in adipocytes. *Molecular Nutrition & Food Research*, 56(12), 1771-1782.

Norman, A. W., Frankel, J. B., Heldt, A. M., & Grodsky, G. M. (1980). Vitamin D deficiency inhibits pancreatic secretion of insulin. *Science*, 209(4458), 823-825.

13 Bao, W., Song, Y., Bertrand, K. A., Tobias, D. K., Olsen, S. F., Chavarro, J. E., ... & Zhang, C. (2018). Prepregnancy habitual intake of vitamin D from diet and supplements in relation to risk of gestational diabetes mellitus: A prospective cohort study: *Journal of Diabetes*, 10(5), 373-379.

14 Ojo, O., Weldon, S. M., Thompson, T., & Vargo, E. J. (2019). The effect of vitamin d supplementation on glycaemic control in women with gestational diabetes mellitus: A systematic review and meta-analysis of randomised controlled trials. *International Journal of Environmental Research and Public Health*, 16(10), 1716.

15 Soheilykhah, S., Mojibian, M., Moghadam, M. J., & Shojaoddiny-Ardekani, A. (2013). The effect of different doses of vitamin D supplementation on insulin resistance during pregnancy. *Gynecological Endocrinology*, 29(4), 396-399.

16 Baynes, H. W., Mideksa, S., & Ambachew, S. (2018). The role of polyunsaturated fatty acids (n-3 PUFAs) on the pancreatic β-cells and insulin action. *Adipocyte*, 7(2), 81-87.

17 Jamilian, M., Samimi, M., Kolahdooz, F., Khalaji, F., Razavi, M., & Asemi, Z. (2016). Omega-3 fatty acid supplementation affects pregnancy outcomes in gestational diabetes: a randomized, double-blind, placebo-controlled trial. *The Journal of Maternal-Fetal & Neonatal Medicine*, 29(4), 669-675.

18 Jamilian, M., Samimi, M., Ebrahimi, F. A., Hashemi, T., Taghizadeh, M., Razavi, M., ... & Asemi, Z. (2017). The effects of vitamin D and omega-3 fatty acid co-supplementation on glycemic control and lipid concentrations in patients with gestational diabetes. *Journal of Clinical Lipidology*, 11(2), 459-468.

19 Xu, J., & Ye, S. (2020). Influence of low-glycemic index diet for gestational diabetes: A meta-analysis of randomized controlled trials. *The Journal of Maternal-Fetal & Neonatal Medicine*, 33(4), 687-692.

Moses, R. G., Barker, M., Winter, M., Petocz, P., & Brand-Miller, J. C. (2009). Can a low–glycemic index diet reduce the need for insulin in gestational diabetes mellitus? A randomized trial. *Diabetes Care*, 32(6), 996-1000.

20 de Barros, M. C., Lopes, M. A., Francisco, R. P., Sapienza, A. D., & Zugaib, M. (2010). Resistance exercise and glycemic control in women with gestational diabetes mellitus. *American Journal of Obstetrics and Gynecology*, 203(6), 556-e1.

21 Louie, J. C. Y., Brand-Miller, J. C., & Moses, R. G. (2013). Carbohydrates, glycemic index, and pregnancy outcomes in gestational diabetes. *Current Diabetes Reports*, 13(1), 6-11.
Moses, R. G., Barker, M., Winter, M., Petocz, P., & Brand-Miller, J. C. (2009). Can a low–glycemic index diet reduce the need for insulin in gestational diabetes mellitus?: A randomized trial. *Diabetes Care*, 32(6), 996-1000.
Wei, J., Heng, W., & Gao, J. (2016). Effects of low glycemic index diets on gestational diabetes mellitus: a meta-analysis of randomized controlled clinical trials. *Medicine*, 95(22).

Chapter 6. Miscarriage Supplements and Progesterone

1 Finley, J., Hay, S., Oldzej, J., Meredith, M. M., Dzidic, N., Slim, R., … & Sahoo, T. (2022). The genomic basis of sporadic and recurrent pregnancy loss: a comprehensive in-depth analysis of 24,900 miscarriages. *Reproductive BioMedicine Online*, 45(1), 125-134.

2 Pérez-Sánchez, C., Aguirre, M. Á., Ruiz-Limón, P., Ábalos-Aguilera, M. C., Jiménez-Gómez, Y., Arias-de la Rosa, I., … & López-Pedrera, C. (2017). Ubiquinol effects on antiphospholipid syndrome prothrombotic profile: a randomized, placebo-controlled trial. *Arteriosclerosis, Thrombosis, and Vascular Biology*, 37(10), 1923-1932.

3 Talukdar, A., Sharma, K. A., Rai, R., Deka, D., & Rao, D. N. (2015). Effect of coenzyme Q10 on Th1/Th2 paradigm in females with idiopathic recurrent pregnancy loss. *American Journal of Reproductive Immunology*, 74(2), 169-180.

4 Noia, G., Littarru, G. P., De Santis, M., Oradei, A., Mastromarino, C., Trivellini, C., & Caruso, A. (1996). Coenzyme Q10 in pregnancy. *Fetal Diagnosis and Therapy*, 11(4), 264-270.

5 Amin, A. F. (2005). N-Acetyl Cysteine (NAC): A possible option in the treatment of unexplained recurrent pregnancy loss. *Fertility and Sterility*, 83(5), S8.
Amin, A. F., Shaaban, O. M., & Bediawy, M. A. (2008). N-acetyl cysteine for treatment of recurrent unexplained pregnancy loss.

Reproductive Biomedicine Online, 17(5), 722–726. https://doi. org/10.1016/s1472-6483(10)60322-7

6   Jang, D. H., Weaver, M. D., & Pizon, A. F. (2013). In vitro study of N-acetylcysteine on coagulation factors in plasma samples from healthy subjects. *Journal of Medical Toxicology,* 9, 49-53. Niemi, T. T., Munsterhjelm, E., Pöyhiä, R., Hynninen, M. S., & Salmenperä, M. T. (2006). The effect of N-acetylcysteine on blood coagulation and platelet function in patients undergoing open repair of abdominal aortic aneurysm. *Blood Coagulation & Fibrinolysis,* 17(1), 29-34.

7   Gupta, S., Agarwal, A., Banerjee, J., & Alvarez, J. G. (2007). The role of oxidative stress in spontaneous abortion and recurrent pregnancy loss: a systematic review. *Obstetrical & Gynecological Survey,* 62(5), 335-347.

8   Dart, R. C., Mullins, M. E., Matoushek, T., Ruha, A. M., Burns, M. M., Simone, K., ... & Rumack, B. H. (2023). Management of Acetaminophen Poisoning in the US and Canada: A Consensus Statement. *JAMA Network Open,* 6(8), e2327739-e2327739.

9   Jenkins, D. D., Wiest, D. B., Mulvihill, D. M., Hlavacek, A. M., Majstoravich, S. J., Brown, T. R., ... & Chang, E. Y. (2016). Fetal and neonatal effects of N-acetylcysteine when used for neuroprotection in maternal chorioamnionitis. *The Journal of Pediatrics,* 168, 67-76. Tenório, M. C. D. S., Graciliano, N. G., Moura, F. A., Oliveira, A. C. M. D., & Goulart, M. O. F. (2021). N-acetylcysteine (NAC): impacts on human health. *Antioxidants,* 10(6), 967. Riggs BS, Bronstein AC, Kulig K, Archer PG, Rumack BH. Acute acetaminophen overdose during pregnancy. *ObstetGynecol* 1989;74(2):247–53. [17] Buhimschi IA, Buhimschi CS,Weiner CP. Protective effect of N-acetylcysteine against fetal death and preterm labor induced by maternal inflammation. *Am JObstetGynecol2003*;188(1):203–8.

10 Shahin, A. Y., Hassanin, I. M., Ismail, A. M., Kruessel, J. S., & Hirchenhain, J. (2009). Effect of oral N-acetyl cysteine on recurrent preterm labor following treatment for bacterial vaginosis. *International Journal of Gynecology & Obstetrics,* 104(1), 44-48.

11 Nyboe Andersen, A., Popovic-Todorovic, B., Schmidt, K. T., Loft, A., Lindhard, A., Højgaard, A., ... & Toft, B. (2002). Progesterone

supplementation during early gestations after IVF or ICSI has no effect on the delivery rates: a randomized controlled trial. *Human Reproduction*, 17(2), 357-361.

Liu, X. R., Mu, H. Q., Shi, Q., Xiao, X. Q., & Qi, H. B. (2012). The optimal duration of progesterone supplementation in pregnant women after IVF/ICSI: a meta-analysis. *Reproductive Biology and Endocrinology*, 10, 1-8.

12 Coomarasamy, A., Devall, A. J., Cheed, V., Harb, H., Middleton, L. J., Gallos, I. D., ... & Jurkovic, D. (2019). A randomized trial of progesterone in women with bleeding in early pregnancy. *New England Journal of Medicine*, 380(19), 1815-1824.

Coomarasamy, A., Williams, H., Truchanowicz, E., Seed, P. T., Small, R., Quenby, S., ... & Rai, R. (2015). A randomized trial of progesterone in women with recurrent miscarriages. *New England Journal of Medicine*, 373(22), 2141-2148.

13 Coomarasamy, A., Devall, A. J., Cheed, V., Harb, H., Middleton, L. J., Gallos, I. D., ... & Jurkovic, D. (2019). A randomized trial of progesterone in women with bleeding in early pregnancy. *New England Journal of Medicine*, 380(19), 1815-1824.

14 Racca, A., Alvarez, M., Garcia Martinez, S., Rodriguez, I., Gonzalez-Foruria, I., Polyzos, N. P., & Coroleu, B. (2023). Assessment of progesterone levels on the day of pregnancy test determination: A novel concept toward individualized luteal phase support. *Frontiers in Endocrinology*, 14, 1090105.

15 Racca, A., Alvarez, M., Garcia Martinez, S., Rodriguez, I., Gonzalez-Foruria, I., Polyzos, N. P., & Coroleu, B. (2023). Assessment of progesterone levels on the day of pregnancy test determination: A novel concept toward individualized luteal phase support. *Frontiers in Endocrinology*, 14, 1090105.

16 Baird, D. D., Weinberg, C. R., McConnaughey, D. R., & Wilcox, A. J. (2003). Rescue of the corpus luteum in human pregnancy. *Biology of Reproduction*, 68(2), 448-456.

Chapter 7. Optimizing Thyroid Function

1 Karcaaltincaba, D., Ozek, M. A., Ocal, N., Calis, P., Inan, M. A., & Bayram, M. (2020). Prevalences of subclinical and overt hypothyroidism with universal screening in early pregnancy. *Archives of Gynecology and Obstetrics*, 301, 681-686.

2   Karcaaltincaba, D., Ozek, M. A., Ocal, N., Calis, P., Inan, M. A., & Bayram, M. (2020). Prevalences of subclinical and overt hypothyroidism with universal screening in early pregnancy. *Archives of Gynecology and Obstetrics*, 301, 681-686.

3   Andersen, S. L., Andersen, S., Vestergaard, P., & Olsen, J. (2018). Maternal thyroid function in early pregnancy and child neurodevelopmental disorders: a Danish nationwide case-cohort study. *Thyroid, 28*(4), 537–546.

Getahun, D., Jacobsen, S. J., Fassett, M. J., Wing, D. A., Xiang, A. H., Chiu, V. Y., & Peltier, M. R. (2018). Association between maternal hypothyroidism and autism spectrum disorders in children. *Pediatric Research, 83*(3), 580.

Nazarpour, S., Tehrani, F. R., Simbar, M., Tohidi, M., Majd, H. A., & Azizi, F. (2017). Effects of levothyroxine treatment on pregnancy outcomes in pregnant women with autoimmune thyroid disease. *European Journal of Endocrinology, 176*(2), 253–265.

4   Adu-Gyamfi, E. A., Wang, Y. X., & Ding, Y. B. (2020). The interplay between thyroid hormones and the placenta: a comprehensive review. *Biology of Reproduction*, 102(1), 8-17.

Silva, J. F., Vidigal, P. N., Galvão, D. D., Boeloni, J. N., Nunes, P. P., Ocarino, N. M., ... & Serakides, R. (2012). Fetal growth restriction in hypothyroidism is associated with changes in proliferative activity, apoptosis and vascularisation of the placenta. *Reproduction, Fertility and Development*, 24(7), 923-931.

5   Silva, J. F., Ocarino, N. M., & Serakides, R. (2014). Maternal thyroid dysfunction affects placental profile of inflammatory mediators and the intrauterine trophoblast migration kinetics. *Reproduction, 147*(6), 803-816.

Vasilopoulou, E., Loubière, L. S., Lash, G. E., Ohizua, O., McCabe, C. J., Franklyn, J. A., ... & Chan, S. Y. (2014). Triiodothyronine regulates angiogenic growth factor and cytokine secretion by isolated human decidual cells in a cell-type specific and gestational age-dependent manner. *Human Reproduction*, 29(6), 1161-1172.

6   Korevaar, T. I., Derakhshan, A., Taylor, P. N., Meima, M., Chen, L., Bliddal, S., ... & Peeters, R. P. (2019). Association of thyroid function test abnormalities and thyroid autoimmunity with preterm birth: a systematic review and meta-analysis. *Jama*, 322(7), 632-641.

Ashoor, G., Maiz, N., Rotas, M., Kametas, N. A., & Nicolaides, K. H. (2010). Maternal thyroid function at 11 to 13 weeks of gestation and subsequent development of preeclampsia. *Prenatal Diagnosis*, 30(11), 1032-1038.

Rao, M., Zeng, Z., Zhou, F., Wang, H., Liu, J., Wang, R., ... & Tang, L. (2019). Effect of levothyroxine supplementation on pregnancy loss and preterm birth in women with subclinical hypothyroidism and thyroid autoimmunity: a systematic review and meta-analysis. *Human Reproduction Update*, 25(3), 344-361.

Tong, Z., Xiaowen, Z., Baomin, C., Aihua, L., Yingying, Z., Weiping, T., & Zhongyan, S. (2016). The effect of subclinical maternal thyroid dysfunction and autoimmunity on intrauterine growth restriction: a systematic review and meta-analysis. *Medicine*, 95(19), e3677.

7 Bein, M., Yu, O. H. Y., Grandi, S. M., Frati, F. Y., Kandil, I., & Filion, K. B. (2021). Levothyroxine and the risk of adverse pregnancy outcomes in women with subclinical hypothyroidism: a systematic review and meta-analysis. *BMC Endocrine Disorders*, 21, 1-17.

Nazarpour, S., Tehrani, F. R., Simbar, M., Tohidi, M., Majd, H. A., & Azizi, F. (2017). Effects of levothyroxine treatment on pregnancy outcomes in pregnant women with autoimmune thyroid disease. *European Journal of Endocrinology, 176*(2), 253–265.

8 Runkle, I., de Miguel, M. P., Barabash, A., Cuesta, M., Diaz, Á., Duran, A., ... & Calle-Pascual, A. (2021). Early levothyroxine treatment for subclinical hypothyroidism or hypothyroxinemia in pregnancy: the st carlos gestational and thyroid protocol. *Frontiers in Endocrinology*, 12, 743057.

9 Nazarpour, S., Tehrani, F. R., Simbar, M., Tohidi, M., Majd, H. A., & Azizi, F. (2017). Effects of levothyroxine treatment on pregnancy outcomes in pregnant women with autoimmune thyroid disease. *European Journal of Endocrinology, 176*(2), 253–265.

10 Hollowell, J. G., & Haddow, J. E. (2007). The prevalence of iodine deficiency in women of reproductive age in the United States of America. *Public Health Nutrition, 10*(12A), 1532–1539.

Lumen, A., & George, N. I. (2017). Estimation of iodine nutrition and thyroid function status in late-gestation pregnant women in the United States: Development and application of a population-based pregnancy model. *Toxicology and Applied Pharmacology, 314*, 24–38.

11 Leung, A. M., & Braverman, L. E. (2014). Consequences of excess iodine. *Nature Reviews Endocrinology, 10*(3), 136.

12 Food Standards Australia and New Zealand (2011). *Advice on brown seaweed for pregnant women; breastfeeding women and children* (27 June 2011). http://www.foodstandards.gov.au/consumer/safety/brownseaweed/Pages/default.aspx

13 Rink, T., Schroth, H. J., Holle, L. H., & Garth, H. (1999). Effect of iodine and thyroid hormones in the induction and therapy of Hashimoto's thyroiditis. *Nuklearmedizin. Nuclear Medicine, 38*(5), 144-149.

Chapter 8. Iron and Anemia

1 Næss-Andresen, M. L., Jenum, A. K., Berg, J. P., Falk, R. S., & Sletner, L. (2023). The impact of recommending iron supplements to women with depleted iron stores in early pregnancy on use of supplements, and factors associated with changes in iron status from early pregnancy to postpartum in a multi-ethnic population-based cohort. *BMC Pregnancy and Childbirth, 23*(1), 1-13.
Hytten, F. (1985). Blood volume changes in normal pregnancy. *Clinics in Haematology, 14*(3), 601–612.

2 Peña-Rosas, J. P., De-Regil, L. M., Dowswell, T., & Viteri, F. E. (2012). Daily oral iron supplementation during pregnancy. *The Cochrane Database of Systematic Reviews, 12*, CD004736.
Næss-Andresen, M. L., Jenum, A. K., Berg, J. P., Falk, R. S., & Sletner, L. (2023). The impact of recommending iron supplements to women with depleted iron stores in early pregnancy on use of supplements, and factors associated with changes in iron status from early pregnancy to postpartum in a multi-ethnic population-based cohort. *BMC Pregnancy and Childbirth, 23*(1), 1-13.

3 Peña-Rosas, J. P., De-Regil, L. M., Dowswell, T., & Viteri, F. E. (2012). Daily oral iron supplementation during pregnancy. *The Cochrane Database of Systematic Reviews, 12*, CD004736.
Thomas, D. G., Kennedy, T. S., Colaizzi, J., Aubuchon-Endsley, N., Grant, S., Stoecker, B., & Duell, E. (2017). Multiple Biomarkers of Maternal Iron Predict Infant Cognitive Outcomes. *Developmental Neuropsychology, 42*(3), 146–159.

Tran, T. D., Biggs, B. A., Tran, T., Simpson, J. A., Hanieh, S., Dwyer, T., & Fisher, J. (2013). Impact on infants' cognitive development of antenatal exposure to iron deficiency disorder and common mental disorders. *Plos One, 8*(9), e74876.

Cusick, S. E., Georgieff, M. K., & Rao, R. (2018). Approaches for reducing the risk of early-life iron deficiency-induced brain dysfunction in children. *Nutrients, 10*(2), 227.

Levy, A., Fraser, D., Katz, M., Mazor, M., & Sheiner, E. (2005). Maternal anemia during pregnancy is an independent risk factor for low birthweight and preterm delivery. *European Journal of Obstetrics & Gynecology and Reproductive Biology, 122*(2), 182–186.

Thomas, D. G., Kennedy, T. S., Colaizzi, J., Aubuchon-Endsley, N., Grant, S., Stoecker, B., & Duell, E. (2017). Multiple Biomarkers of Maternal Iron Predict Infant Cognitive Outcomes. *Developmental Neuropsychology, 42*(3), 146–159.

4   Georgieff, M. K. (2023). The importance of iron deficiency in pregnancy on fetal, neonatal, and infant neurodevelopmental outcomes. *International Journal of Gynecology & Obstetrics*, 162, 83-88.

5   Georgieff, M. K. (2023). The importance of iron deficiency in pregnancy on fetal, neonatal, and infant neurodevelopmental outcomes. *International Journal of Gynecology & Obstetrics*, 162, 83-88.

6   Tamura, T., Goldenberg, R. L., Hou, J., Johnston, K. E., Cliver, S. P., Ramey, S. L., & Nelson, K. G. (2002). Cord serum ferritin concentrations and mental and psychomotor development of children at five years of age. *The Journal of Pediatrics*, 140(2), 165-170.

Riggins, T., Miller, N. C., Bauer, P. J., Georgieff, M. K., & Nelson, C. A. (2009). Consequences of low neonatal iron status due to maternal diabetes mellitus on explicit memory performance in childhood. *Developmental Neuropsychology*, 34(6), 762-779.

Christian P, Murray-Kolb LE, Khatry SK, et al. Prenatal micronutrient supplementation and intellectual and motor function in early school-aged children in Nepal. *JAMA*. 2010;304:2716-2723.

7   Georgieff, M. K. (2023). The importance of iron deficiency in pregnancy on fetal, neonatal, and infant neurodevelopmental

outcomes. *International Journal of Gynecology & Obstetrics*, 162, 83-88.

8   Auerbach, M., Abernathy, J., Juul, S., Short, V., & Derman, R. (2021). Prevalence of iron deficiency in first trimester, nonanemic pregnant women. The Journal of Maternal-Fetal & Neonatal Medicine, 34(6), 1002-1005.

9   Auerbach, M. (2023). Optimizing diagnosis and treatment of iron deficiency and iron deficiency anemia in women and girls of reproductive age: Clinical opinion. *International Journal of Gynecology & Obstetrics*, 162, 68-77.

10   Auerbach, M. (2023). Optimizing diagnosis and treatment of iron deficiency and iron deficiency anemia in women and girls of reproductive age: Clinical opinion. *International Journal of Gynecology & Obstetrics*, 162, 68-77

11   Milman, N., Jønsson, L., Dyre, P., Pedersen, P. L., & Larsen, L. G. (2014). Ferrous bisglycinate 25 milligrams iron is as effective as ferrous sulfate 50 milligrams iron in the prophylaxis of iron deficiency and anemia during pregnancy in a randomized trial. *Journal of Perinatal Medicine, 42*(2), 197–206.

12   Milman, N., Jønsson, L., Dyre, P., Pedersen, P. L., & Larsen, L. G. (2014). Ferrous bisglycinate 25 milligrams iron is as effective as ferrous sulfate 50 milligrams iron in the prophylaxis of iron deficiency and anemia during pregnancy in a randomized trial. *Journal of Perinatal Medicine, 42*(2), 197–206.

13   Maeda, Y., Ogawa, K., Morisaki, N., Tachibana, Y., Horikawa, R., & Sago, H. (2020). Association between perinatal anemia and postpartum depression: A prospective cohort study of Japanese women. *International Journal of Gynecology & Obstetrics*, 148(1), 48-52.

14   Maeda, Y., Ogawa, K., Morisaki, N., Tachibana, Y., Horikawa, R., & Sago, H. (2020). Association between perinatal anemia and postpartum depression: A prospective cohort study of Japanese women. *International Journal of Gynecology & Obstetrics*, 148(1), 48-52.

15   Wassef, A., Nguyen, Q. D., & St-André, M. (2019). Anaemia and depletion of iron stores as risk factors for postpartum depression: a literature review. *Journal of Psychosomatic Obstetrics & Gynecology*, 40(1), 19-28.

Chapter 9. Prenatal Testing

1   Lo, Y. D., Corbetta, N., Chamberlain, P. F., Rai, V., Sargent, I. L., Redman, C. W., & Wainscoat, J. S. (1997). Presence of fetal DNA in maternal plasma and serum. *The Lancet*, 350(9076), 485-487.

2   Li, C., Xiong, M., Zhan, Y., Zhang, J., Qiao, G., Li, J., & Yang, H. (2023). Clinical Potential of Expanded Noninvasive Prenatal Testing for Detection of Aneuploidies and Microdeletion/ Microduplication Syndromes. *Molecular Diagnosis & Therapy*, 27(6), 769-779.

3   Bussolaro, S., Raymond, Y. C., Acreman, M. L., Guido, M., Costa, F. D. S., Rolnik, D. L., & Fantasia, I. (2023). The accuracy of prenatal cell-free DNA screening for sex chromosome abnormalities: A systematic review and meta-analysis. *American Journal of Obstetrics & Gynecology MFM*, 5(3), 100844

4   Li, C., Xiong, M., Zhan, Y., Zhang, J., Qiao, G., Li, J., & Yang, H. (2023). Clinical Potential of Expanded Noninvasive Prenatal Testing for Detection of Aneuploidies and Microdeletion/ Microduplication Syndromes. *Molecular Diagnosis & Therapy*, 27(6), 769-779.

5   Gross, S. J., Stosic, M., McDonald-McGinn, D. M., Bassett, A. S., Norvez, A., Dhamankar, R., … & Benn, P. (2016). Clinical experience with single-nucleotide polymorphism-based non-invasive prenatal screening for 22q11. 2 deletion syndrome. *Ultrasound in Obstetrics & Gynecology*, 47(2), 177-183.

6   Scott, F., Smet, M. E., Elhindi, J., Mogra, R., Sunderland, L., Ferreira, A., … & McLennan, A. (2023). Late first-trimester ultrasound findings can alter management after high-risk NIPT result. *Ultrasound in Obstetrics & Gynecology*.

7   Smith, K., Lowther, G., Maher, E., Hourihan, T., Wilkinson, T., & Wolstenholme, J. (1999). The predictive value of findings of the common aneuploidies, trisomies 13, 18 and 21, and numerical sex chromosome abnormalities at CVS: experience from the ACC UK collaborative study. Prenatal Diagnosis: Published in Affiliation with the International Society for Prenatal Diagnosis, 19(9), 817-826.

8   Schuring-Blom, G. H., Boer, K., Knegt, A. C., Verjaal, M., & Leschot, N. J. (2002). Trisomy 13 or 18 (mosaicism) in first trimester cytotrophoblast cells: false-positive results in 11 out

of 51 cases. *European Journal of Obstetrics & Gynecology and Reproductive Biology*, 101(2), 161-168.

9   Salomon, L. J., Sotiriadis, A., Wulff, C. B., Odibo, A., & Akolekar, R. (2019). Risk of miscarriage following amniocentesis or chorionic villus sampling: systematic review of literature and updated meta-analysis. *Ultrasound in Obstetrics & Gynecology*, 54(4), 442-451.

10 Madjunkov, M., Abramov, R., Glass, K. B., Baratz, A. Y., Sharma, P. A., Madjunkova, S., & Librach, C. L. (2023). Noninvasive prenatal testing (NIPT) after euploid embryo transfer shows high concordance with PGT-A results and low NIPT predictive values. *Fertility and Sterility*, 120(4), e50.

Chapter 10. Letting Go of Worry and Finding Joy

1   Seppälä, E. M., Bradley, C., Moeller, J., Harouni, L., Nandamudi, D., & Brackett, M. A. (2020). Promoting mental health and psychological thriving in university students: a randomized controlled trial of three well-being interventions. *Frontiers in Psychiatry*, 590.

2   Balban, M. Y., Neri, E., Kogon, M. M., Weed, L., Nouriani, B., Jo, B., ... & Huberman, A. D. (2023). Brief structured respiration practices enhance mood and reduce physiological arousal. *Cell Reports Medicine*, 4(1).

3   Arch, J. J., & Craske, M. G. (2006). Mechanisms of mindfulness: Emotion regulation following a focused breathing induction. *Behaviour Research and Therapy*, 44(12), 1849-1858.

4   Seppälä, E. M., Nitschke, J. B., Tudorascu, D. L., Hayes, A., Goldstein, M. R., Nguyen, D. T., ... & Davidson, R. J. (2014). Breathing-based meditation decreases posttraumatic stress disorder symptoms in US Military veterans: A randomized controlled longitudinal study. *Journal of Traumatic Stress*, 27(4), 397-405.

5   Al-Kaleel, A., Al-Gailani, L., Demir, M., & Aygün, H. (2022). Vitamin D may prevent COVID-19 induced pregnancy complication. *Medical Hypotheses*, 158, 110733.

6   Hughes, L. M., Schuler, A., Sharmuk, M., Schauer, J. M., Pavone, M. E., & Bernardi, L. A. (2022). Early β-hCG levels predict live birth after single embryo transfer. *Journal of Assisted Reproduction and Genetics*, 39(10), 2355-2364.

7   Ahmed, S. R., El-Sammani, M. E. K., Al-Sheeha, M. A. A.,
    Aitallah, A. S., & Khan, F. J. (2012). Pregnancy outcome in women
    with threatened miscarriage: a year study. *Materia Socio-Medica*,
    24(1), 26.
8   Christiansen, O. B. (2014). Recurrent miscarriage is a useful
    and valid clinical concept. *Acta Obstetricia et Gynecologica
    Scandinavica*, 93(9), 852-857.
9   Vlaanderen, W. (2014). Is recurrent miscarriage a useful clinical
    concept?. *Acta Obstetricia et Gynecologica Scandinavica*, 93(9),
    848-851.

Chapter 11. Managing Pregnancy Nausea

1   Fejzo, M. S., Sazonova, O. V., Sathirapongsasuti, J. F.,
    Hallgrímsdóttir, I. B., Vacic, V., MacGibbon, K. W., ... &
    Mullin, P. M. (2018). Placenta and appetite genes GDF15 and
    IGFBP7 are associated with hyperemesis gravidarum. *Nature
    Communications*, 9(1), 1178.
    Fejzo, M. S., MacGibbon, K. W., First, O., Quan, C., & Mullin, P. M.
    (2022). Whole-exome sequencing uncovers new variants in GDF15
    associated with hyperemesis gravidarum. *BJOG: An International
    Journal of Obstetrics & Gynaecology*, 129(11), 1845-1852.
2   Andersson-Hall, U., Joelsson, L., Svedin, P., Mallard, C., &
    Holmäng, A. (2021). Growth-differentiation-factor 15 levels in
    obese and healthy pregnancies: relation to insulin resistance and
    insulin secretory function. *Clinical Endocrinology*, 95(1), 92-100.
3   Andersson-Hall, U., Joelsson, L., Svedin, P., Mallard, C., &
    Holmäng, A. (2021). Growth-differentiation-factor 15 levels in
    obese and healthy pregnancies: relation to insulin resistance and
    insulin secretory function. *Clinical Endocrinology*, 95(1), 92-100.
    Sjøberg, K. A., Sigvardsen, C. M., Alvarado-Diaz, A., Andersen,
    N. R., Larance, M., Seeley, R. J., ... & Richter, E. A. (2023). GDF15
    increases insulin action in the liver and adipose tissue via a
    β-adrenergic receptor-mediated mechanism. *Cell Metabolism*,
    35(8), 1327-1340.
4   Fejzo, M., Rocha, N., Cimino, I., Lockhart, S. M., Petry, C. J., Kay,
    R. G., ... & O'Rahilly, S. (2024). GDF15 linked to maternal risk of
    nausea and vomiting during pregnancy. *Nature*, 625(7996), 760-767.

5   Fejzo, M., Rocha, N., Cimino, I., Lockhart, S. M., Petry, C. J., Kay, R. G., ... & O'Rahilly, S. (2024). GDF15 linked to maternal risk of nausea and vomiting during pregnancy. *Nature*, 625(7996), 760-767.

6   Fejzo, M., Rocha, N., Cimino, I., Lockhart, S. M., Petry, C. J., Kay, R. G., ... & O'Rahilly, S. (2024). GDF15 linked to maternal risk of nausea and vomiting during pregnancy. *Nature*, 625(7996), 760-767.

7   Yilmaz, H., Cakmak, M., Darcin, T., Inan, O., Bilgic, M. A., Bavbek, N., & Akcay, A. (2016). Can serum Gdf-15 be associated with functional Iron deficiency in hemodialysis patients?. *Indian Journal of Hematology and Blood Transfusion*, 32, 221-227. Lockhart, S. M., Saudek, V., & O'Rahilly, S. (2020). GDF15: a hormone conveying somatic distress to the brain. *Endocrine Reviews*, 41(4), bnaa007.

8   Miyaue, N., Yabe, H., & Nagai, M. (2020). Serum growth differentiation factor 15 levels and clinical manifestations in patients with thiamine deficiency. *Neurology and Clinical Neuroscience*, 8(5), 245-250.

9   Miyaue, N., Yabe, H., & Nagai, M. (2020). Serum growth differentiation factor 15 levels and clinical manifestations in patients with thiamine deficiency. *Neurology and Clinical Neuroscience*, 8(5), 245-250.

10 Lockhart, S. M., Saudek, V., & O'Rahilly, S. (2020). GDF15: a hormone conveying somatic distress to the brain. *Endocrine Reviews*, 41(4), bnaa007.

11 Schernthaner-Reiter, M. H., Kasses, D., Tugendsam, C., Riedl, M., Peric, S., Prager, G., ... & Vila, G. (2016). Growth differentiation factor 15 increases following oral glucose ingestion: effect of meal composition and obesity. *European Journal of Endocrinology*, 175(6), 623-631.

12 Dormuth, C. R., Winquist, B., Fisher, A., Wu, F., Reynier, P., Suissa, S., ... & Paterson, J. M. (2021). Comparison of pregnancy outcomes of patients treated with ondansetron vs alternative antiemetic medications in a multinational, population-based cohort. *JAMA Network Open*, 4(4), e215329-e215329.

13 Hinkle, S. N., Mumford, S. L., Grantz, K. L., Silver, R. M., Mitchell, E. M., Sjaarda, L. A., ... & Schisterman, E. F. (2016). Association of nausea and vomiting during pregnancy with pregnancy loss: a secondary analysis of a randomized clinical trial. *JAMA Internal Medicine*, 176(11), 1621-1627.

14 Lacroix, R., Eason, E., & Melzack, R. (2000). Nausea and vomiting during pregnancy: a prospective study of its frequency, intensity, and patterns of change. American journal of obstetrics and gynecology, 182(4), 931-937.

Chapter 12. The Big Nutrition Controversies

1   Mills, J.L.; Holmes, L.B.; Aarons, J.H.; Simpson, J.L.; Brown, Z.A.; Jovanovic-Peterson, L.G.; Conley, M.R.; Graubard, B.I.; Knopp, R.H.; Metzger, B.E. Moderate caffeine use and the risk of spontaneous abortion and intrauterine growth retardation. *J. Am. Med. Assoc.* 1993, 269, 593–597.
    Klebanoff, M. A., Levine, R. J., DerSimonian, R., Clemens, J. D., & Wilkins, D. G. (1999). Maternal serum paraxanthine, a caffeine metabolite, and the risk of spontaneous abortion. *New England Journal of Medicine*, 341(22), 1639-1644.
    Savitz, D.A.; Chan, R.L.; Herring, A.H.; Howards, P.P.; Hartmann, K.E. Caffeine and miscarriage risk. *Epidemiology* 2008, 19, 55–62.
    Bech, B.H.; Obel, C.; Henriksen, T.B.; Olsen, J. Effect of reducing caffeine intake on birth weight and length of gestation: Randomised controlled trial. *BMJ* 2007, 334, 409.
    Clausson, B.; Granath, F.; Ekbom, A.; Lundgren, S.; Nordmark, A.; Signorello, L.B.; Cnattingius, S. Effect of caffeine exposure during pregnancy on birth weight and gestational age. *Am. J. Epidemiol.* 2002, 155, 429–436.
2   Heazell, A. E., Timms, K., Scott, R. E., Rockliffe, L., Budd, J., Li, M., … & Thompson, J. M. (2021). Associations between consumption of coffee and caffeinated soft drinks and late stillbirth—Findings from the Midland and North of England stillbirth case-control study. *European Journal of Obstetrics & Gynecology and Reproductive Biology*, 256, 471-477.
    Chen, L. W., Wu, Y., Neelakantan, N., Chong, M. F. F., Pan, A., & van Dam, R. M. (2016). Maternal caffeine intake during pregnancy and risk of pregnancy loss: a categorical and dose–response meta-analysis of prospective studies. *Public Health Nutrition*, 19(7), 1233-1244.
    Greenwood, D. C., Thatcher, N. J., Ye, J., Garrard, L., Keogh, G., King, L. G., & Cade, J. E. (2014). Caffeine intake during pregnancy and adverse birth outcomes: a systematic review and

dose–response meta-analysis. *European Journal of Epidemiology*, 29, 725-734.

Greenwood, D. C., Alwan, N., Boylan, S., Cade, J. E., Charvill, J., Chipps, K. C., ... & Wild, C. P. (2010). Caffeine intake during pregnancy, late miscarriage and stillbirth. *European Journal of Epidemiology*, 25, 275-280.

Signorello, L. B., Nordmark, A., Granath, F., Blot, W. J., McLaughlin, J. K., Anneren, G., ... & Cnattingius, S. (2001). Caffeine metabolism and the risk of spontaneous abortion of normal karyotype fetuses. *Obstetrics & Gynecology*, 98(6), 1059-1066.

3 Weng, X., Odouli, R., & Li, D. K. (2008). Maternal caffeine consumption during pregnancy and the risk of miscarriage: a prospective cohort study. American journal of obstetrics and gynecology, 198(3), 279-e1.

4 Hoyt AT, Browne M, Richardson S, et al. Maternal caffeine consumption and small for gestational age births: results from a population-based case-control study. *Matern Child Health J* 2014;18:1540–51

Chen L-W, Fitzgerald R, Murrin CM, et al. Associations of maternal caffeine intake with birth outcomes: results from the Lifeways cross generation cohort study. *Am J Clin Nutr* 2018;108:1301–8.

Kobayashi S, Sata F, Murata K, et al. Dose-dependent associations between prenatal caffeine consumption and small for gestational age, preterm birth, and reduced birthweight in the Japan Environment and Children's Study. *Paediatr Perinat Epidemiol* 2019;33:185–94.

Modzelewska D, Bellocco R, Elfvin A, et al. Caffeine exposure during pregnancy, small for gestational age birth and neonatal outcome – results from the Norwegian Mother and Child Cohort Study. *BMC Pregnancy Childbirth* 2019;19:80.

Bakker R, Steegers EAP, Obradov A, et al. Maternal caffeine intake from coffee and tea, fetal growth, and the risks of adverse birth outcomes: the generation R study. *Am J Clin Nutr* 2010;91:1691–8.

Sengpiel V, Elind E, Bacelis J, et al. Maternal caffeine intake during pregnancy is associated with birth weight but not with gestational length: results from a large prospective observational cohort study. *BMC Med* 2013;11:42.

Bech BH, Frydenberg M, Henriksen TB, et al. Coffee consumption during pregnancy and birth weight: does smoking modify the association? *J Caffeine Res* 2015;5:65–72.

Rhee J, Kim R, Kim Y, et al. Maternal caffeine consumption during pregnancy and risk of low birth weight: a dose-response meta-analysis of observational studies. *PLoS One.* 2015;10(7):e0132334.

Chen L-W, Wu Y, Neelakantan N, Chong MF-F, Pan A, van Dam RM. Maternal caffeine intake during pregnancy is associated with risk of low birth weight: a systematic review and dose-response meta-analysis. *BMC Med.* 2014;12(1):174.

5   Fortier, I., Marcoux, S., & Beaulac-Baillargeon, L. (1993). Relation of caffeine intake during pregnancy to intrauterine growth retardation and preterm birth. *American Journal of Epidemiology*, 137(9), 931-940.

CARE Study Group. (2008). Maternal caffeine intake during pregnancy and risk of fetal growth restriction: a large prospective observational study. *The* BMJ, 337.

Soltani, S., Salari-Moghaddam, A., Saneei, P., Askari, M., Larijani, B., Azadbakht, L., & Esmaillzadeh, A. (2022). Maternal caffeine consumption during pregnancy and risk of low birth weight: a dose–response meta-analysis of cohort studies. *Critical Reviews in Food Science and Nutrition*, 63(2), 224-233.

Jin, F., & Qiao, C. (2021). Association of maternal caffeine intake during pregnancy with low birth weight, childhood overweight, and obesity: a meta-analysis of cohort studies. *International Journal of Obesity*, 45(2), 279-287.

6   Askari, M., Bazshahi, E., Payande, N., Mobaderi, T., Fahimfar, N., & Azadbakht, L. (2023). Relationship between caffeine intake and small for gestational age and preterm birth: a dose-response meta-analysis. *Critical Reviews in Food Science and Nutrition*, 1-11.

7   Bech B H, Obel C, Henriksen T B, Olsen J. Effect of reducing caffeine intake on birth weight and length of gestation: randomised controlled trial *BMJ* 2007; 334 :409

8   Gleason, J. L., Tekola-Ayele, F., Sundaram, R., Hinkle, S. N., Vafai, Y., Louis, G. M. B., ... & Grantz, K. L. (2021). Association between maternal caffeine consumption and metabolism and neonatal anthropometry: A secondary analysis of the NICHD fetal growth studies–singletons. *JAMA Network Open*, 4(3), e213238-e213238.

9   Kesmodel, U. S., Bertrand, J., Støvring, H., Skarpness, B., Denny, C. H., Mortensen, E. L., & Lifestyle During Pregnancy Study Group. (2012). The effect of different alcohol drinking patterns in early to mid pregnancy on the child's intelligence, attention, and executive function. *BJOG: An International Journal of Obstetrics & Gynaecology*, 119(10), 1180-1190.

10 Astley, S., & Grant, T. (2012). Another perspective on 'The effect of different alcohol drinking patterns in early to mid-pregnancy on the child's intelligence, attention, and executive function'. *BJOG: An International Journal of Obstetrics and Gynaecology*, 119(13), 1672-1672.

11 Lees, B., Mewton, L., Jacobus, J., Valadez, E. A., Stapinski, L. A., Teesson, M., … & Squeglia, L. M. (2020). Association of prenatal alcohol exposure with psychological, behavioral, and neurodevelopmental outcomes in children from the adolescent brain cognitive development study. *American Journal of Psychiatry*, 177(11), 1060-1072.
    Long, X., & Lebel, C. (2022). Evaluation of brain alterations and behavior in children with low levels of prenatal alcohol exposure. *JAMA Network Open*, 5(4), e225972-e225972.

12 Long, X., & Lebel, C. (2022). Evaluation of brain alterations and behavior in children with low levels of prenatal alcohol exposure. *JAMA Network Open*, 5(4), e225972-e225972.

13 Endrikat, S., Gallagher, D., Pouillot, R., Quesenberry, H. H., Labarre, D., Schroeder, C. M., & Kause, J. (2010). A comparative risk assessment for Listeria monocytogenes in prepackaged versus retail-sliced deli meat. *Journal of Food Protection*, 73(4), 612-619.

14 Endrikat, S., Gallagher, D., Pouillot, R., Quesenberry, H. H., Labarre, D., Schroeder, C. M., & Kause, J. (2010). A comparative risk assessment for Listeria monocytogenes in prepackaged versus retail-sliced deli meat. *Journal of Food Protection*, 73(4), 612-619.

Chapter 13. Minimizing Toxins and Finding Balance

1   Mostafalou, S., & Abdollahi, M. (2017). Pesticides: an update of human exposure and toxicity. Archives of toxicology, 91(2), 549-599.

2   Hertz-Picciotto, I., Sass, J. B., Engel, S., Bennett, D. H., Bradman, A., Eskenazi, B., … & Whyatt, R. (2018). Organophosphate exposures during pregnancy and child neurodevelopment:

Recommendations for essential policy reforms. PLoS medicine, 15(10), e1002671.

3   Roberts, J. R., & Karr, C. J. (2012). Pesticide exposure in children. Pediatrics, peds-2012.

4   El-Salam, M. A., Hegazy, A. A., Elhady, M., Ibrahim, G. E., & Hussein, R. (2017). Biomarkers of Organophosphate Pesticides and Attention-Deficit/Hyperactivity Disorder in Children: A Case-Control Study. J Environ Anal Toxicol, 7(460), 2161-0525.
Roberts, J. R., Dawley, E. H., & Reigart, J. R. (2018). Children's low-level pesticide exposure and associations with autism and ADHD: a review. Pediatric research, 1.
Schmidt, R. J., Kogan, V., Shelton, J. F., Delwiche, L., Hansen, R. L., Ozonoff, S., ... & Tancredi, D. (2018, February). Combined Exposures to Prenatal Pesticides and Folic Acid Intake in Relation to Autism Spectrum Disorder. In ISEE Conference Abstracts.
Roberts, J. R., & Karr, C. J. (2012). Pesticide exposure in children. Pediatrics, peds-2012.

5   Jenkins, H. M., Meeker, J. D., Zimmerman, E., Cathey, A., Fernandez, J., Montañez, G. H., ... & Watkins, D. J. (2024). Gestational glyphosate exposure and early childhood neurodevelopment in a Puerto Rico birth cohort. Environmental Research, 246, 118114.

6   Myers, J. P., Antoniou, M. N., Blumberg, B., Carroll, L., Colborn, T., Everett, L. G., ... & Vandenberg, L. N. (2016). Concerns over use of glyphosate-based herbicides and risks associated with exposures: a consensus statement. Environmental Health, 15(1), 19

7   Myers, J. P., Antoniou, M. N., Blumberg, B., Carroll, L., Colborn, T., Everett, L. G., ... & Vandenberg, L. N. (2016). Concerns over use of glyphosate-based herbicides and risks associated with exposures: a consensus statement. Environmental Health, 15(1), 19

8   Temkin, A. (2018) Breakfast With a Dose of Roundup. Environmental Working Group. https://www.ewg.org/childrenshealth/glyphosateincereal/

9   Yang, T., Doherty, J., Zhao, B., Kinchla, A. J., Clark, J. M., & He, L. (2017). Effectiveness of commercial and homemade washing agents in removing pesticide residues on and in apples. Journal of agricultural and food chemistry, 65(44), 9744-9752.

10   Brown University. News from Brown - Joseph Braun. https://news.brown.edu/new-faculty/life-sciences/joseph-braun

11 Tewar, S., Auinger, P., Braun, J. M., Lanphear, B., Yolton, K., Epstein, J. N., ... & Froehlich, T. E. (2016). Association of bisphenol A exposure and attention-deficit/hyperactivity disorder in a national sample of US children. Environmental research, 150, 112-118.

Hong, S. B., Hong, Y. C., Kim, J. W., Park, E. J., Shin, M. S., Kim, B. N., ... & Cho, S. C. (2013). Bisphenol A in relation to behavior and learning of school-age children. Journal of child psychology and psychiatry, 54(8), 890-899.

Harley, K. G., Gunier, R. B., Kogut, K., Johnson, C., Bradman, A., Calafat, A. M., & Eskenazi, B. (2013). Prenatal and early childhood bisphenol A concentrations and behavior in school-aged children. Environmental research, 126, 43-50

Perera, F., Vishnevetsky, J., Herbstman, J. B., Calafat, A. M., Xiong, W., Rauh, V., & Wang, S. (2012). Prenatal bisphenol a exposure and child behavior in an inner-city cohort. Environmental health perspectives, 120(8), 1190.

Roen, E. L., Wang, Y., Calafat, A. M., Wang, S., Margolis, A., Herbstman, J., ... & Perera, F. P. (2015). Bisphenol A exposure and behavioral problems among inner city children at 7–9 years of age. Environmental research, 142, 739-745.

12 Braun, J. M., Kalkbrenner, A. E., Calafat, A. M., Bernert, J. T., Ye, X., Silva, M. J., ... & Lanphear, B. P. (2010). Variability and predictors of urinary bisphenol A concentrations during pregnancy. Environmental health perspectives, 119(1), 131-137.

13 Ragusa, A., Svelato, A., Santacroce, C., Catalano, P., Notarstefano, V., Carnevali, O., ... & Giorgini, E. (2021). Plasticenta: First evidence of microplastics in human placenta. Environment international, 146, 106274.

Hunt, K., Davies, A., Fraser, A., Burden, C., Howell, A., Buckley, K., ... & Bakhbakhi, D. (2024). Exposure to microplastics and human reproductive outcomes: A systematic review. BJOG: An International Journal of Obstetrics & Gynaecology, 131(5), 675-683.

14 Siwakoti, R. C., Cathey, A., Ferguson, K. K., Hao, W., Cantonwine, D. E., Mukherjee, B., ... & Meeker, J. D. (2023). Prenatal per-and polyfluoroalkyl substances (PFAS) exposure in relation to preterm birth subtypes and size-for-gestational age in the LIFECODES cohort 2006–2008. Environmental research, 237, 116967.

Meng, Q., Inoue, K., Ritz, B., Olsen, J., & Liew, Z. (2018). Prenatal Exposure to Perfluoroalkyl Substances and Birth Outcomes; An Updated Analysis from the Danish National Birth Cohort. International journal of environmental research and public health, 15(9), 1832.

Manzano-Salgado, C. B., Casas, M., Lopez-Espinosa, M. J., Ballester, F., Iñiguez, C., Martinez, D., ... & Sunyer, J. (2017). Prenatal exposure to perfluoroalkyl substances and birth outcomes in a Spanish birth cohort. Environment international, 108, 278-284.

Woods, M. M., Lanphear, B. P., Braun, J. M., & McCandless, L. C. (2017). Gestational exposure to endocrine disrupting chemicals in relation to infant birth weight: a Bayesian analysis of the HOME Study. Environmental Health, 16(1), 115.

15 Ghassabian, A., Bell, E. M., Ma, W. L., Sundaram, R., Kannan, K., Louis, G. M. B., & Yeung, E. (2018). Concentrations of perfluoroalkyl substances and bisphenol A in newborn dried blood spots and the association with child behavior. Environmental Pollution

Zhou, Y., Li, Q., Wang, P., Li, J., Zhao, W., Zhang, L., ... & Zhang, Y. (2023). Associations of prenatal PFAS exposure and early childhood neurodevelopment: Evidence from the Shanghai Maternal-Child Pairs Cohort. Environment International, 173, 107850.

16 Meuwly, R., Brunner, K., Fragnière, C., Sager, F., & Dudler, V. (2005). Heat stability and migration from silicone baking moulds. Mitteilungen aus Lebensmitteluntersuchung und Hygiene, 96(5), 281.

17 Soni, M. G., White, S. M., Flamm, W. G., & Burdock, G. A. (2001). Safety evaluation of dietary aluminum. Regulatory toxicology and Pharmacology, 33(1), 66-79.

18 Swan SH, Main KM, Liu F, Stewart SL, Kruse RL, Calafat AM, Mao CS, Redmon JB, Ternand CL, Sullivan S, Teague JL; Study for Future Families Research Team.Decrease in anogenital distance among male infants with prenatal phthalateexposure. Environ Health Perspect. 2005 Aug;113(8):1056-61. Erratum in: Environ Health Perspect. 2005 Sep;113(9):A583. ("Swan 2005").

Swan SH. Environmental phthalate exposure in relation to reproductive outcomes and other health endpoints in humans. Environ Res. 2008 Oct; 108(2):177-84.

Foster, P. M. (2006). Disruption of reproductive development in male rat offspring following in utero exposure to phthalate esters. International journal of andrology, 29(1), 140-147.

Howdeshell KL, Wilson VS, Furr J, Lambright CR, Rider CV, Blystone CR, Hotchkiss AK, Gray LE Jr. A mixture of five phthalate esters inhibits fetal testicular testosterone production in the sprague-dawley rat in a cumulative, dose-additive manner. Toxicol Sci. 2008 Sep;105(1):153-65.

Akingbemi BT, Ge R, Klinefelter GR, Zirkin BR, Hardy MP. Phthalate-induced Leydig cell hyperplasia is associated with multiple endocrine disturbances. Proc Natl Acad Sci U S A. 2004 Jan 20;101(3):775-80

Borch J, Ladefoged O, Hass U, Vinggaard AM. Steroidogenesis in fetal male rats is reduced by DEHP and DINP, but endocrine effects of DEHP are not modulated by DEHA in fetal, prepubertal and adult male rats. Reprod Toxicol. 2004 Jan-Feb;18(1):53-61;

Klinefelter GR, Laskey JW, Winnik WM, Suarez JD, Roberts NL, Strader LF, Riffle BW, Veeramachaneni DN. Novel molecular targets associated with testicular dysgenesis induced by gestational exposure to diethylhexyl phthalate in the rat: a role for estradiol. Reproduction. 2012 Dec; 144(6):747-61

Latini G, et al. In utero exposure to di-(2-ethylhexyl)phthalate and duration of human pregnancy. Environmental Health Perspectives. 2003;111:1783–1785.

19 Latini G, et al. In utero exposure to di-(2-ethylhexyl)phthalate and duration of human pregnancy. Environmental Health Perspectives. 2003;111:1783–1785.

Meeker JD, Hu H, Cantonwine DE, Lamadrid-Figueroa H, Calafat AM, Ettinger AS, Hernandez-Avila M, Loch-Caruso R, Téllez-Rojo MM. Urinary phthalate metabolites in relation to preterm birth in Mexico city. Environ. Health Perspect. 2009;117(10):1587–1592.

Whyatt RM, Adibi JJ, Calafat AM, Camann DE, Rauh V, Bhat HK, Perera FP, Andrews H, Just AC, Hoepner L, Tang D, Hauser R. Prenatal di(2-ethylhexyl) phthalate exposure and length of gestation among an inner-city cohort. Pediatrics. 2009;124(6):e1213–e1220.

Meeker JD, Hu H, Cantonwine DE, Lamadrid-Figueroa H, Calafat AM, Ettinger AS, Hernandez-Avila M, Loch-Caruso R, Téllez-Rojo MM. Urinary phthalate metabolites in relation to preterm birth in Mexico city. Environ. Health Perspect. 2009;117(10):1587–1592.

20 Latini G, Del Vecchio A, Massaro M, Verrotti A, De Felice C. In utero exposure to phthalates and fetal development. Curr Med Chem. 2006;13:2527–2534.

Ferguson, K. K., Chen, Y. H., VanderWeele, T. J., McElrath, T. F., Meeker, J. D., & Mukherjee, B. (2016). Mediation of the relationship between maternal phthalate exposure and preterm birth by oxidative stress with repeated measurements across pregnancy. Environmental health perspectives, 125(3), 488-494.

21 Olesen, T. S., Bleses, D., Andersen, H. R., Grandjean, P., Frederiksen, H., Trecca, F., ... & Andersson, A. M. (2018). Prenatal phthalate exposure and language development in toddlers from the Odense Child Cohort. Neurotoxicology and teratology, 65, 34-41.

Bornehag, C. G., Lindh, C., Reichenberg, A., Wikström, S., Hallerback, M. U., Evans, S. F., ... & Swan, S. H. (2018). Association of Prenatal Phthalate Exposure With Language Development in Early Childhood. JAMA pediatrics.

Whyatt RM, Liu X, Rauh VA, Calafat AM, Just AC, Hoepner L, Diaz D, Quinn J, Adibi J, Perera FP, Factor-Litvak P. Maternal prenatal urinary phthalate metabolite concentrations and child mental, psychomotor, and behavioral development at 3 years of age. Environ Health Perspect 2012;120:290

Yolton K, Xu Y, Strauss D, Altaye M, Calafat AM, Khoury J. Prenatal exposure to bisphenol A and phthalates and infant neurobehavior. Neurotoxicol Teratol 2011;33:558-66;

Engel SM, Zhu C, Berkowitz GS, Calafat AM, Silva MJ, Miodovnik A, Wolff MS. Prenatal phthalate exposure and performance on the Neonatal Behavioral Assessment Scale in a multiethnic birth cohort. Neurotoxicology 2009;30:522-8;

Kim Y, Ha EH, Kim EJ, Park H, Ha M, Kim JH, Hong YC, Chang N, Kim BN. Prenatal exposure to phthalates and infant development at 6 months: prospective Mothers and Children's Environmental Health (MOCEH) study. Environ Health Perspect 2011;119:1495-500;

Engel SM, Miodovnik A, Canfield RL, Zhu C, Silva MJ, Calafat AM, Wolff MS. Prenatal phthalate exposure is associated with childhood behavior and executive functioning. Environ Health Perspect 2010;118:565-71;

Swan SH, Liu F, Hines M, Kruse RL, Wang C, Redmon JB, Sparks A, Weiss B. Prenatal phthalate exposure and reduced masculine play in boys. Int J Androl 2010;33:259-69;

Miodovnik A, Engel SM, Zhu C, Ye X, Soorya LV, Silva MJ, Calafat AM, Wolff MS. Endocrine disruptors and childhood social impairment. Neurotoxicology 2011;32:261-7;

Factor-Litvak, P., Insel, B., Calafat, A. M., Liu, X., Perera, F., Rauh, V. A., & Whyatt, R. M. (2014). Persistent associations between maternal prenatal exposure to phthalates on child IQ at age 7 years. PloS one, 9(12), e114003.

Braun, J. M. (2017). Early-life exposure to EDCs: role in childhood obesity and neurodevelopment. Nature Reviews Endocrinology, 13(3), 161.

Kobrosly, R. W., Evans, S., Miodovnik, A., Barrett, E. S., Thurston, S. W., Calafat, A. M., & Swan, S. H. (2014). Prenatal phthalate exposures and neurobehavioral development scores in boys and girls at 6–10 years of age. Environmental health perspectives, 122(5), 521.

Olesen, T. S., Bleses, D., Andersen, H. R., Grandjean, P., Frederiksen, H., Trecca, F., ... & Andersson, A. M. (2018). Prenatal phthalate exposure and language development in toddlers from the Odense Child Cohort. Neurotoxicology and teratology, 65, 34-41.

Bornehag, C. G., Lindh, C., Reichenberg, A., Wikström, S., Hallerback, M. U., Evans, S. F., ... & Swan, S. H. (2018). Association of Prenatal Phthalate Exposure With Language Development in Early Childhood. JAMA pediatrics.

22 Zota, A. R., Calafat, A. M., & Woodruff, T. J. (2014). Temporal trends in phthalate exposures: findings from the National Health and Nutrition Examination Survey, 2001–2010. Environmental health perspectives, 122(3), 235-241.

Göen, T., Dobler, L., Koschorreck, J., Müller, J., Wiesmüller, G. A., Drexler, H., & Kolossa-Gehring, M. (2011). Trends of the internal phthalate exposure of young adults in Germany—follow-up of a retrospective human biomonitoring study. International journal of hygiene and environmental health, 215(1), 36-45.

23 Koch, H. M., Lorber, M., Christensen, K. L., Pälmke, C., Koslitz, S., & Brüning, T. (2013). Identifying sources of phthalate exposure

with human biomonitoring: results of a 48 h fasting study with urine collection and personal activity patterns. International journal of hygiene and environmental health, 216(6), 672-681.

Zota, A. R., Phillips, C. A., & Mitro, S. D. (2016). Recent fast food consumption and bisphenol A and phthalates exposures among the US population in NHANES, 2003-2010. Environmental health perspectives, 124(10), 1521. http://kleanupkraft.org/PhthalatesLabReport.pdf

24 http://kleanupkraft.org/PhthalatesLabReport.pdf
Rabin, R. C. (2017). The Chemicals in Your Mac and Cheese. New York Times.

25 Rabin, R. C. (2017). The Chemicals in Your Mac and Cheese. New York Times

26 Rudel RA, Gray JM, Engel CL, Rawsthorne TW, Dodson RE, Ackerman JM, Rizzo J, Nudelman JL, Brody JG. Food packaging and bisphenol A and bis(2-ethyhexyl) phthalate exposure: findings from a dietary intervention. Environ Health Perspect. 2011 Jul;119(7):914-20.

27 Cao, X. L., Zhao, W., Churchill, R., & Hilts, C. (2014). Occurrence of di-(2-ethylhexyl) adipate and phthalate plasticizers in samples of meat, fish, and cheese and their packaging films. Journal of food protection, 77(4), 610-620

28 Wittassek M, Koch HM, Angerer J, Bruning T. Assessing exposure to phthalates – the human biomonitoring approach. Mol Nutr Food Res. 2011;55:7–31

29 Jiang, Y., Zhao, H., Xia, W., Li, Y., Liu, H., Hao, K., ... & Peng, Y. (2019). Prenatal exposure to benzophenones, parabens and triclosan and neurocognitive development at 2 years. Environment international, 126, 413-421.
Kawaguchi, M., Morohoshi, K., Imai, H., Morita, M., Kato, N., & Himi, T. (2010). Maternal exposure to isobutyl-paraben impairs social recognition in adult female rats. Experimental animals, 59(5), 631-635.
Ali, E. H., & Elgoly, A. H. M. (2013). Combined prenatal and postnatal butyl paraben exposure produces autism-like symptoms in offspring: comparison with valproic acid autistic model. Pharmacology Biochemistry and Behavior, 111, 102-110.

30 Wang, X., Ouyang, F., Feng, L., Wang, X., Liu, Z., & Zhang, J. (2017). Maternal urinary triclosan concentration in relation to

maternal and neonatal thyroid hormone levels: a prospective study. Environmental health perspectives, 125(6), 067017.

31 Ghazipura, M., McGowan, R., Arslan, A., & Hossain, T. (2017). Exposure to benzophenone-3 and reproductive toxicity: a systematic review of human and animal studies. Reproductive Toxicology, 73, 175-183.
Environmental Working Group (2018). The Trouble With Ingredients in Sunscreens. https://www.ewg.org/sunscreen/report/the-trouble-with-sunscreen-chemicals/

32 Chien, A. L., Qi, J., Rainer, B., Sachs, D. L., & Helfrich, Y. R. (2016). Treatment of acne in pregnancy. J Am Board Fam Med, 29(2), 254-262.

Chapter 14. Exercises for an Easier Pregnancy and Recovery

1 Mogren, I. M., & Pohjanen, A. I. (2005). Low back pain and pelvic pain during pregnancy: prevalence and risk factors. *Spine*, 30(8), 983-991.

2 Lynders, C. (2019). The critical role of development of the transversus abdominis in the prevention and treatment of low back pain. *HSS Journal*®, 15(3), 214-220.
Richardson, C. A., Snijders, C. J., Hides, J. A., Damen, L., Pas, M. S., & Storm, J. (2002). The relation between the transversus abdominis muscles, sacroiliac joint mechanics, and low back pain. *Spine*, 27(4), 399-405.

3 Ghandali, N. Y., Iravani, M., Habibi, A., & Cheraghian, B. (2021). The effectiveness of a Pilates exercise program during pregnancy on childbirth outcomes: a randomised controlled clinical trial. *BMC Pregnancy and Childbirth*, 21(1), 1-11.
Rodríguez-Blanque, R., Sánchez-García, J. C., Sánchez-López, A. M., & Aguilar-Cordero, M. J. (2019). Physical activity during pregnancy and its influence on delivery time: a randomized clinical trial. *PeerJ*, 7, e6370.
Watkins, V. Y., O'Donnell, C. M., Perez, M., Zhao, P., England, S., Carter, E. B., ... & Raghuraman, N. (2021). The impact of physical activity during pregnancy on labor and delivery. *American Journal of Obstetrics and Gynecology*, 225(4), 437-e1.

4 Rodríguez-Blanque, R., Sánchez-García, J. C., Sánchez-López, A. M., & Aguilar-Cordero, M. J. (2019). Physical activity during

pregnancy and its influence on delivery time: a randomized clinical trial. *PeerJ*, 7, e6370.

5   Chiarello, C. M., Falzone, L. A., McCaslin, K. E., Patel, M. N., & Ulery, K. R. (2005). The effects of an exercise program on diastasis recti abdominis in pregnant women. *The Journal of Women's & Pelvic Health Physical Therapy*, 29(1), 11-16.

6   Chiarello, C. M., Falzone, L. A., McCaslin, K. E., Patel, M. N., & Ulery, K. R. (2005). The effects of an exercise program on diastasis recti abdominis in pregnant women. *The Journal of Women's & Pelvic Health Physical Therapy*, 29(1), 11-16.

7   Chiarello, C. M., Falzone, L. A., McCaslin, K. E., Patel, M. N., & Ulery, K. R. (2005). The effects of an exercise program on diastasis recti abdominis in pregnant women. *The Journal of Women's & Pelvic Health Physical Therapy*, 29(1), 11-16.

8   Couper, S., Clark, A., Thompson, J. M., Flouri, D., Aughwane, R., David, A. L., ... & Stone, P. R. (2021). The effects of maternal position, in late gestation pregnancy, on placental blood flow and oxygenation: an MRI study. *The Journal of Physiology*, 599(6), 1901-1915.

Chapter 15. Pregnancy Vaccine Decisions

1   Bourdeau, M., Vadlamudi, N. K., Bastien, N., Embree, J., Halperin, S. A., Jadavji, T., ... & Pernica, J. (2023). Pediatric RSV-Associated Hospitalizations Before and During the COVID-19 Pandemic. *JAMA Network Open*, 6(10), e2336863-e2336863.

2   Fleming-Dutra, K. E. (2023). Use of the Pfizer respiratory syncytial virus vaccine during pregnancy for the prevention of respiratory syncytial virus–associated lower respiratory tract disease in infants: recommendations of the Advisory Committee on Immunization Practices—United States, 2023. MMWR. *Morbidity and Mortality Weekly Report*, 72.

3   Fleming-Dutra, K. E. (2023). Use of the Pfizer respiratory syncytial virus vaccine during pregnancy for the prevention of respiratory syncytial virus–associated lower respiratory tract disease in infants: recommendations of the Advisory Committee on Immunization Practices—United States, 2023. MMWR. *Morbidity and Mortality Weekly Report*, 72.

4   Fleming-Dutra, K. E. (2023). Use of the Pfizer respiratory syncytial virus vaccine during pregnancy for the prevention of

respiratory syncytial virus–associated lower respiratory tract disease in infants: recommendations of the Advisory Committee on Immunization Practices—United States, 2023. MMWR. *Morbidity and Mortality Weekly Report*, 72.

5   Kampmann, B., Madhi, S. A., Munjal, I., Simões, E. A., Pahud, B. A., Llapur, C., ... & Gurtman, A. (2023). Bivalent prefusion F vaccine in pregnancy to prevent RSV illness in infants. *New England Journal of Medicine*, 388(16), 1451-1464.

6   D. Mertz, C.K. Lo, L. Lytvyn, J.R. Ortiz, M. Loeb, I. Flurisk, Pregnancy as a risk factor for severe influenza infection: an individual participant data meta-analysis *BMC Infect Dis*, 19 (1) (2019), p. 683
    Mazagatos, C., Delgado-Sanz, C., Oliva, J., Gherasim, A., Larrauri, A., & Spanish Influenza Surveillance System. (2018). Exploring the risk of severe outcomes and the role of seasonal influenza vaccination in pregnant women hospitalized with confirmed influenza, Spain, 2010/11-2015/16. *Plos One*, 13(8), e0200934.

7   Mølgaard-Nielsen, D., Fischer, T. K., Krause, T. G., & Hviid, A. (2019). Effectiveness of maternal immunization with trivalent inactivated influenza vaccine in pregnant women and their infants. *Journal of Internal Medicine*, 286(4), 469-480.
    Regan, A. K., De Klerk, N., Moore, H. C., Omer, S. B., Shellam, G., & Effler, P. V. (2016). Effectiveness of seasonal trivalent influenza vaccination against hospital-attended acute respiratory infections in pregnant women: a retrospective cohort study. *Vaccine*, 34(32), 3649-3656.
    Thompson, M. G., Kwong, J. C., Regan, A. K., Katz, M. A., Drews, S. J., Azziz-Baumgartner, E., ... & Simmonds, K. (2018). Influenza Vaccine Effectiveness in Preventing Influenza-associated Hospitalizations During Pregnancy: A Multi-country Retrospective Test Negative Design Study, 2010–2016. *Clinical Infectious Diseases*.

8   Mølgaard-Nielsen, D., Fischer, T. K., Krause, T. G., & Hviid, A. (2019). Effectiveness of maternal immunization with trivalent inactivated influenza vaccine in pregnant women and their infants. *Journal of Internal Medicine*, 286(4), 469-480.
    Duque, J., Howe, A. S., Azziz-Baumgartner, E., & Petousis-Harris, H. (2023). Multi-decade national cohort identifies adverse pregnancy and birth outcomes associated with acute respiratory

illness hospitalisations during the influenza season. *Influenza and Other Respiratory Viruses*, 17(1), e13063.

9   Munoz, F. M. (2012). Safety of influenza vaccines in pregnant women. *American Journal of Obstetrics and Gynecology*, 207(3), S33-S37.

Håberg, S. E., Trogstad, L., Gunnes, N., Wilcox, A. J., Gjessing, H. K., Samuelsen, S. O., ... & Madsen, S. (2013). Risk of fetal death after pandemic influenza virus infection or vaccination. *New England Journal of Medicine, 368*(4), 333–340.

Moro, P. L., Broder, K., Zheteyeva, Y., Walton, K., Rohan, P., Sutherland, A., ... & Vellozzi, C. (2011). Adverse events in pregnant women following administration of trivalent inactivated influenza vaccine and live attenuated influenza vaccine in the Vaccine Adverse Event Reporting System, 1990-2009. *American Journal of Obstetrics and Gynecology, 204*(2), 146–e1.

Tamma, P. D., Ault, K. A., del Rio, C., Steinhoff, M. C., Halsey, N. A., & Omer, S. B. (2009). Safety of influenza vaccination during pregnancy. *American Journal of Obstetrics and Gynecology*, 201(6), 547-552.

WHO. World Health Organization Global Advisory Committee on Vaccine Safety. Safety of immunization during pregnancy. A review of the evidence (2014) Available from: https://www.who.int/vaccine_safety/publications/safety_pregnancy_nov2014.pdf

10 Zerbo, O., Qian, Y., Yoshida, C., Fireman, B. H., Klein, N. P., & Croen, L. A. (2017). Association between influenza infection and vaccination during pregnancy and risk of autism spectrum disorder. *JAMA Pediatrics, 171*(1), e163609–e163609.

11 Becerra-Culqui, T. A., Getahun, D., Chiu, V., Sy, L. S., & Tseng, H. F. (2022). Prenatal influenza vaccination or influenza infection and autism spectrum disorder in offspring. *Clinical Infectious Diseases*, 75(7), 1140-1148.

Ludvigsson, J. F., Winell, H., Sandin, S., Cnattingius, S., Stephansson, O., & Pasternak, B. (2020). Maternal influenza A (H1N1) immunization during pregnancy and risk for autism spectrum disorder in offspring: a cohort study. *Annals of Internal Medicine*, 173(8), 597-604.

12 Centers for Disease Control (2016), *Create a Circle of Protection Around Babies*, https://www.cdc.gov/vaccines/pregnancy/family-caregivers/index.html

Eick, A. A., Uyeki, T. M., Klimov, A., Hall, H., Reid, R., Santosham, M., & O'brien, K. L. (2011). Maternal influenza vaccination and effect on influenza virus infection in young infants. *Archives of Pediatrics & Adolescent Medicine, 165*(2), 104–111.

13 Zhong Z, Haltalli M, Holder B, Rice T, Donaldson B, O' Driscoll M, Le-Doare K, Kampmann B, Tregoning JS. The impact of timing of maternal influenza immunization on infant antibody levels at birth. *Clin Exp Immunol.* 2019;195:139–52.

14 Shakib, J. H., Korgenski, K., Presson, A. P., Sheng, X., Varner, M. W., Pavia, A. T., & Byington, C. L. (2016). Influenza in infants born to women vaccinated during pregnancy. *Pediatrics*, e20152360.

15 Sahni, L. C., Olson, S. M., Halasa, N. B., Stewart, L. S., Michaels, M. G., Williams, J. V., … & New Vaccine Surveillance Network Collaborators. (2023). Maternal Vaccine Effectiveness Against Influenza-Associated Hospitalizations and Emergency Department Visits in Infants. *JAMA Pediatrics.*
Mølgaard-Nielsen, D., Fischer, T. K., Krause, T. G., & Hviid, A. (2019). Effectiveness of maternal immunization with trivalent inactivated influenza vaccine in pregnant women and their infants. *Journal of Internal Medicine*, 286(4), 469-480.

16 Aydillo, T., Balsera-Manzanero, M., Rojo-Fernandez, A., Escalera, A., Salamanca-Rivera, C., Pachón, J., … & Cordero, E. (2024). Concomitant administration of seasonal influenza and COVID-19 mRNA vaccines. *Emerging Microbes & Infections,* 13(1), 2292068.
Xie, Z., Hamadi, H. Y., Mainous, A. G., & Hong, Y. R. (2023). Association of dual COVID-19 and seasonal influenza vaccination with COVID-19 infection and disease severity. *Vaccine*, 41(4), 875-878.

17 Villar, J., Conti, C. P. S., Gunier, R. B., Ariff, S., Craik, R., Cavoretto, P. I., … & Papageorghiou, A. T. (2023). Pregnancy outcomes and vaccine effectiveness during the period of omicron as the variant of concern, INTERCOVID-2022: a multinational, observational study. *The Lancet*, 401(10375), 447-457.
Rahmati, M., Yon, D. K., Lee, S. W., Butler, L., Koyanagi, A., Jacob, L., … & Smith, L. (2023). Effects of COVID-19 vaccination during pregnancy on SARS-CoV-2 infection and maternal and neonatal outcomes: A systematic review and meta-analysis. *Reviews in Medical Virology*, 33(3), e2434.

18 Baxter, R., Bartlett, J., Fireman, B., Lewis, E., & Klein, N. P. (2017). Effectiveness of vaccination during pregnancy to prevent infant pertussis. *Pediatrics*, e20164091.

19 Naidu, M. A., Muljadi, R., Davies-Tuck, M. L., Wallace, E. M., & Giles, M. L. (2016). The optimal gestation for pertussis vaccination during pregnancy: a prospective cohort study. *American Journal of Obstetrics and Gynecology*, 215(2), 237-e1.

20 Peterson, J.T.; Zareba, A.M.; Fitz-Patrick, D.; Essink, B.J.; Scott, D.A.; Swanson, K.A.; Chelani, D.; Radley, D.; Cooper, D.; Jansen, K.U.; et al. Safety and Immunogenicity of a Respiratory Syncytial Virus Prefusion F Vaccine When Coadministered with a Tetanus, Diphtheria, and Acellular Pertussis Vaccine. *J. Infect. Dis.* 2022, 225, 2077–2086.

21 Vásquez-Procopio, J., Torres-Torres, J., Borboa-Olivares, H., Sosa, S. E. Y., Martínez-Portilla, R. J., Solis-Paredes, M., ... & Estrada-Gutierrez, G. (2022). Association between 25-OH Vitamin D Deficiency and COVID-19 Severity in Pregnant Women. *International Journal of Molecular Sciences*, 23(23), 15188.

22 Seven, B., Gunduz, O., Ozgu-Erdinc, A. S., Sahin, D., Moraloglu Tekin, O., & Keskin, H. L. (2022). Correlation between 25-hydroxy vitamin D levels and COVID-19 severity in pregnant women: a cross-sectional study. *The Journal of Maternal-Fetal & Neonatal Medicine*, 35(25), 8817-8822.

Al-Kaleel, A., Al-Gailani, L., Demir, M., & Aygün, H. (2022). Vitamin D may prevent COVID-19 induced pregnancy complication. *Medical Hypotheses*, 158, 110733.

Sinaci, S., Ocal, D. F., Yetiskin, D. F. Y., Hendem, D. U., Buyuk, G. N., Ayhan, S. G., ... & Sahin, D. (2021). Impact of vitamin D on the course of COVID-19 during pregnancy: A case control study. *The Journal of Steroid Biochemistry and Molecular Biology*, 213, 105964.

Mazaheri-Tehrani, S., Mirzapour, M. H., Yazdi, M., Fakhrolmobasheri, M., & Abhari, A. P. (2022). Serum vitamin D levels and COVID-19 during pregnancy: A systematic review and meta-analysis. *Clinical Nutrition ESPEN*.

23 Spinato G, Fabbris C, Costantini G, Conte F, Scotton PG, Cinetto F, et al. The effect of isotonic saline nasal lavages in improving symptoms in SARS-CoV-2 infection: A Case-Control Study. *Front Neurol.* (2021) 12:794471. doi: 10.3389/fneur.2021.794471

24 Chatterjee U, Chakraborty A, Naskar S, Saha B, Bandyapadhyay B, Shee S. Efficacy of normal saline nasal spray and gargle on SARS-CoV-2 for prevention of COVID-19 pneumonia. *Res Square.* (2021). PPR277214. doi: 10.21203/rs.3.rs-153598/v2

25 Baxter, A. L., Schwartz, K. R., Johnson, R. W., Kuchinski, A. M., Swartout, K. M., Srinivasa Rao, A. S., ... & Schwartz, R. (2022). Rapid initiation of nasal saline irrigation to reduce severity in high-risk COVID+ outpatients. *Ear, Nose & Throat Journal,* 01455613221123737.

26 Huijghebaert, S., Parviz, S., Rabago, D., Baxter, A., Chatterjee, U., Khan, F. R., ... & Hsu, S. (2023). Saline nasal irrigation and gargling in COVID-19: a multidisciplinary review of effects on viral load, mucosal dynamics, and patient outcomes. *Frontiers in Public Health*, 11, 1161881.

27 Parviz S, Duncan L, Rabago D. Soap and water to hands and face-eye rinse, nasal irrigation and gargling with saline for COVID-19 with anecdotal evidence. *Rhinology.* (2021) 4:185-93. doi: 10.4193/RHINOL/21.040
Gutiérrez-García R, De la Cerda-Ángeles JC, Cabrera-Licona A, Delgado-Enciso I, Mervitch-Sigal N, Paz-Michel BA. Nasopharyngeal and oropharyngeal rinses with neutral electrolyzed water prevents COVID-19 in front-line health professionals: a randomized, open-label, controlled trial in a general hospital in Mexico City. *Biomed Rep.* (2022) 16:11. doi: 10.3892/br.2021.1494
Yilmaz YZ, Yilmaz BB, Ozdemir YE, Kocazeybek BS, Karaali R, Çakan D, et al. Effects of hypertonic alkaline nasal irrigation on COVID-19. *Laryngoscope Investig Otolaryngol.* (2021) 6:1240–7. doi: 10.1002/lio2.686

28 Ramalingam S, Graham C, Dove J, Morrice L, Sheikh A. A pilot, open labelled, randomised controlled trial of hypertonic saline nasal irrigation and gargling for the common cold. *Sci Rep.* 2019;9(1):1015.

Chapter 16. Third-Trimester Monitoring and Induction

1 Tveit, J. V. H., Saastad, E., Stray-Pedersen, B., Børdahl, P. E., Flenady, V., Fretts, R., & Frøen, J. F. (2009). Reduction of late stillbirth with the introduction of fetal movement information

and guidelines–a clinical quality improvement. BMC pregnancy and childbirth, 9, 1-10.

2   https://countthekicks.org/why-we-count/evidence/

3   Burn, S. C., Yao, R., Diaz, M., Rossi, J., & Contag, S. (2022). Impact of labor induction at 39 weeks gestation compared with expectant management on maternal and perinatal morbidity among a cohort of low-risk women. *The Journal of Maternal-Fetal & Neonatal Medicine*, 35(25), 9208-9214.

4   Rath, W., & Wolff, F. (2014). Increased risk of stillbirth in older mothers—a rationale for induction of labour before term?. *Zeitschrift fur Geburtshilfe und Neonatologie*, 218(5), 190-194.

5   Pay, A. S. D., Wiik, J., Backe, B., Jacobsson, B., Strandell, A., & Klovning, A. (2015). Symphysis-fundus height measurement to predict small-for-gestational-age status at birth: a systematic review. *BMC pregnancy and Childbirth*, 15(1), 1-9.
    Sparks, T. N., Cheng, Y. W., McLaughlin, B., Esakoff, T. F., & Caughey, A. B. (2011). Fundal height: a useful screening tool for fetal growth?. *The Journal of Maternal-Fetal & Neonatal Medicine*, 24(5), 708-712.

6   Niknafs, P., & Sibbald, J. (2001). Accuracy of single ultrasound parameters in detection of fetal growth restriction. *American Journal of Perinatology*, 18(06), 325-334.
    Caradeux, J., Martinez-Portilla, R. J., Peguero, A., Sotiriadis, A., & Figueras, F. (2019). Diagnostic performance of third-trimester ultrasound for the prediction of late-onset fetal growth restriction: a systematic review and meta-analysis. *American Journal of Obstetrics and Gynecology*, 220(5), 449-459.

7   Hofmeyr, G. J., Gülmezoglu, A. M., Novikova, N., & Cochrane Pregnancy and Childbirth Group. (1996). Maternal hydration for increasing amniotic fluid volume in oligohydramnios and normal amniotic fluid volume. *Cochrane Database of Systematic Reviews*, 2012(2).
    Flack, N. J., Sepulveda, W., Bower, S., & Fisk, N. M. (1995). Acute maternal hydration in third-trimester oligohydramnios: effects on amniotic fluid volume, uteroplacental perfusion, and fetal blood flow and urine output. *American Journal of Obstetrics and Gynecology*, 173(4), 1186-1191.

8   Gizzo, S., Noventa, M., Vitagliano, A., Dall'Asta, A., D'Antona, D., Aldrich, C. J., ... & Patrelli, T. S. (2015). An update on

maternal hydration strategies for amniotic fluid improvement in isolated oligohydramnios and normohydramnios: evidence from a systematic review of literature and meta-analysis. *PloS One*, 10(12), e0144334.

9   Fait, G., Pauzner, D., Gull, I., Lessing, J. B., Jaffa, A. J., & Wolman, I. (2003). Effect of 1 week of oral hydration on the amniotic fluid index. *The Journal of Reproductive Medicine*, 48(3), 187-190.

10 Buscicchio, G., Lorenzi, S., & Tranquilli, A. L. (2013). The effects of different concentrations of cocoa in the chocolate intaken by the mother on fetal heart rate. *The Journal of Maternal-Fetal & Neonatal Medicine*, 26(15), 1465-1467.
    Hasanpour, S., Raouf, S., Shamsalizadeh, N., Bani, S., Ghojazadeh, M., & Sheikhan, F. (2013). Evaluation of the effects of acoustic stimulation and feeding mother stimulation on non-reactive non-stress test: a randomized clinical trial. *Archives of Gynecology and Obstetrics*, 287, 1105-1110.

11 Dolker, H. E., & Basar, F. (2019). The effect of music on the non-stress test and maternal anxiety. *Complementary Therapies in Clinical Practice*, 35, 259-264.

12 American College of Obstetricians and Gynecologists, Committee on Obstetric Practice, & Society for Maternal-Fetal Medicine. (2021). Indications for outpatient antenatal fetal surveillance: ACOG Committee Opinion, Number 828. *Obstetrics and Gynecology*, 137(6), e177-e197.
    Fox, N. S., Rebarber, A., Silverstein, M., Roman, A. S., Klauser, C. K., & Saltzman, D. H. (2013). The effectiveness of antepartum surveillance in reducing the risk of stillbirth in patients with advanced maternal age. *European Journal of Obstetrics & Gynecology and Reproductive Biology*, 170(2), 387-390.
    Solmonovich, R., Blitz, M. J., Alvarez, A., & Goldman, R. H. (2023). FETAL INDICATIONS FOR INDUCTION OF LABOR AMONG IVF AND NON-IVF NTSV (NULLIPAROUS, TERM, SINGLETON, VERTEX) PREGNANCIES. *Fertility and Sterility*, 120(4), e326.

13 https://medicine.yale.edu/obgyn/kliman/placenta/epv/

14 Thompson, B. B., Holzer, P. H., & Kliman, H. J. (2024). Placental pathology findings in unexplained pregnancy losses. *Reproductive Sciences*, 31(2), 488-504.

Murdaugh, K. L., & Florescue, H. (2023). Small estimated placental volume (EPV) in the setting of decreased fetal movement. *Clinical Imaging*, 104, 110027.

15 Zhou, C. G., Frank, Z. C., & Caughey, A. B. (2019). 538: Outcomes of elective induction of labor at 39 weeks versus expectant management until week 40. *American Journal of Obstetrics & Gynecology*, 220(1), S359-S360.

16 Hedegaard, M., Lidegaard, Ø., Skovlund, C. W., Mørch, L. S., & Hedegaard, M. (2014). Reduction in stillbirths at term after new birth induction paradigm: results of a national intervention. *BMJ Open*, 4(8), e005785.
    Lidegaard, Ø., Krebs, L., Petersen, O. B. B., Damm, N. P., & Tabor, A. (2020). Are the Danish stillbirth rates still record low? A nationwide ecological study. *BMJ Open*, 10(12), e040716.
    Grobman, W. A., Rice, M. M., Reddy, U. M., Tita, A. T., Silver, R. M., Mallett, G., ... & Macones, G. A. (2018). Labor induction versus expectant management in low-risk nulliparous women. *New England Journal of Medicine*, 379(6), 513-523.

17 Sengupta, S., Carrion, V., Shelton, J., Wynn, R. J., Ryan, R. M., Singhal, K., & Lakshminrusimha, S. (2013). Adverse neonatal outcomes associated with early-term birth. *JAMA Pediatrics*, 167(11), 1053-1059.
    Hibbard, J. U., Wilkins, I., Sun, L., Gregory, K., Haberman, S., Hoffman, M., ... & Zhang, J. (2010). Respiratory morbidity in late preterm births. *JAMA*, 304(4), 419-425.

18 Clark SL , Miller DD , Belfort MA , Dildy GA , Frye DK , Meyers JA . Neonatal and maternal outcomes associated with elective term delivery . *Am J Obstet Gynecol* 2009 ; 200 : 156.e1 – 4

19 Lindquist, A., Hastie, R., Kennedy, A., Gurrin, L., Middleton, A., Quach, J., ... & Tong, S. (2022). Developmental outcomes for children after elective birth at 39 weeks' gestation. *JAMA Pediatrics*, 176(7), 654-663.
    Wehby, G. L. (2023). Association Between Gestational Age and Academic Achievement of Children Born at Term. *JAMA Network Open*, 6(7), e2326451-e2326451.

20 Grobman, W. A., Rice, M. M., Reddy, U. M., Tita, A. T., Silver, R. M., Mallett, G., ... & Macones, G. A. (2018). Labor induction versus expectant management in low-risk nulliparous women. *New England Journal of Medicine*, 379(6), 513-523.

21 Hong, J., Atkinson, J., Mitchell, A. R., Tong, S., Walker, S. P., Middleton, A., … & Hastie, R. (2023). Comparison of maternal labor-related complications and neonatal outcomes following elective induction of labor at 39 weeks of gestation vs expectant management: a systematic review and meta-analysis. *JAMA Network Open*, 6(5), e2313162-e2313162.

Namath, A., Vazquez, D., Pollak, Y., Banner, G., & Haider, S. (2023). INDUCTION OF LABOR AND IVF: DOES ARRIVE APPLY?. *Fertility and Sterility*, 120(1), e11-e12.

Fonseca, M. J., Santos, F., Afreixo, V., Silva, I. S., & do Céu Almeida, M. (2020). Does induction of labor at term increase the risk of cesarean section in advanced maternal age? A systematic review and meta-analysis. *European Journal of Obstetrics & Gynecology and Reproductive Biology*, 253, 213-219.

22 Hong, J., Atkinson, J., Mitchell, A. R., Tong, S., Walker, S. P., Middleton, A., … & Hastie, R. (2023). Comparison of maternal labor-related complications and neonatal outcomes following elective induction of labor at 39 weeks of gestation vs expectant management: a systematic review and meta-analysis. *JAMA Network Open*, 6(5), e2313162-e2313162.

23 Carbone, L., De Vivo, V., Saccone, G., D'Antonio, F., Mercorio, A., Raffone, A., … & Zullo, F. (2019). Sexual intercourse for induction of spontaneous onset of labor: a systematic review and meta-analysis of randomized controlled trials. *The Journal of Sexual Medicine*, 16(11), 1787-1795.

Singh, N., Tripathi, R., Mala, Y. M., & Yedla, N. (2014). Breast stimulation in low-risk primigravidas at term: does it aid in spontaneous onset of labour and vaginal delivery? A pilot study. *BioMed Research International*, 2014.

24 Pereira, I. B., Silva, R., Ayres-de-Campos, D., & Clode, N. (2022). Physical exercise at term for enhancing the spontaneous onset of labor: a randomized clinical trial. *The Journal of Maternal-Fetal & Neonatal Medicine*, 35(4), 775-779

Chapter 17. Delivery Decisions

1 Hollister, N., Todd, C., Ball, S., Thorp-Jones, D., & Coghill, J. (2012). Minimising the risk of accidental dural puncture with epidural analgesia for labour: a retrospective review of risk factors. *International Journal of Obstetric Anesthesia*, 21(3), 236-241.

2   Ohel, G., Gonen, R., Vaida, S., Barak, S., & Gaitini, L. (2006). Early versus late initiation of epidural analgesia in labor: does it increase the risk of cesarean section? A randomized trial. I, 194(3), 600-605.

3   Zhang, J., Yancey, M. K., Klebanoff, M. A., Schwarz, J., & Schweitzer, D. (2001). Does epidural analgesia prolong labor and increase risk of cesarean delivery? A natural experiment. I, 185(1), 128-134.

4   Navarro-Tapia, E., Sebastiani, G., Sailer, S., Almeida Toledano, L., Serra-Delgado, M., García-Algar, Ó., & Andreu-Fernández, V. (2020). Probiotic supplementation during the perinatal and infant period: effects on gut dysbiosis and disease. Nutrients, 12(8), 2243.

5   Azad, M. B., Konya, T., Persaud, R. R., Guttman, D. S., Chari, R. S., Field, C. J., ... & Becker, A. B. (2016). Impact of maternal intrapartum antibiotics, method of birth and breastfeeding on gut microbiota during the first year of life: a prospective cohort study. *BJOG: An International Journal of Obstetrics & Gynaecology, 123*(6), 983–993.

6   Thomas, P., & Margulis, J. (2016). The Vaccine-friendly Plan: Dr. Paul's Safe and Effective Approach to Immunity and Health-from Pregnancy Through Your Child's Teen Years. Ballantine Books.

7   Petricevic, L., Unger, F. M., Viernstein, H., & Kiss, H. (2008). Randomized, double-blind, placebo-controlled study of oral lactobacilli to improve the vaginal flora of postmenopausal women. *European Journal of Obstetrics & Gynecology and Reproductive Biology, 141*(1), 54–57.
Anukam, K. C., Osazuwa, E., Osemene, G. I., Ehigiagbe, F., Bruce, A. W., & Reid, G. (2006). Clinical study comparing probiotic Lactobacillus GR-1 and RC-14 with metronidazole vaginal gel to treat symptomatic bacterial vaginosis. *Microbes and Infection, 8*(12-13), 2772–2776.
Martinez, R. C. R., Franceschini, S. A., Patta, M. C., Quintana, S. M., Candido, R. C., Ferreira, J. C., ... & Reid, G. (2009). Improved treatment of vulvovaginal candidiasis with fluconazole plus probiotic Lactobacillus rhamnosus GR-1 and Lactobacillus reuteri RC-14. *Letters in Applied Microbiology, 48*(3), 269–274.

8   Ho, M., Chang, Y. Y., Chang, W. C., Lin, H. C., Wang, M. H., Lin, W. C., & Chiu, T. H. (2016). Oral Lactobacillus rhamnosus GR-1 and Lactobacillus reuteri RC-14 to reduce group B Streptococcus

colonization in pregnant women: a randomized controlled trial. *Taiwanese Journal of Obstetrics and Gynecology, 55*(4), 515–518.

9   Sharpe M, Shah V, Freire-Lizama T, et al.. Effectiveness of oral intake of lactobacillus rhamnosus GR-1 and lactobacillus reuteri RC-14 on group B streptococcus colonization during pregnancy: a midwifery-led double-blind randomized controlled pilot trial. *J Matern Fetal Neonatal Med* 2021;34:1814–21.

Olsen P, Williamson M, Traynor V, et al.. The impact of oral probiotics on vaginal group B streptococcal colonisation rates in pregnant women: a pilot randomised control study. *Women Birth* 2018;31:31–7.

10 McDonald, S. J., & Middleton, P. (2008). Effect of timing of umbilical cord clamping of term infants on maternal and neonatal outcomes. *Cochrane Database Syst Rev, 2*(2), CD004074.

Salcido, C., Shahidi, S. A., Poeltler, D. M., Gollin, Y., Johnston, L. A., & Katheria, A. C. (2023). Maternal bleeding complications and neonatal outcomes following early versus delayed umbilical cord clamping in cesarean deliveries for very low birthweight infants. *Journal of Perinatology, 43*(1), 39-43.

11 Ashish, K. C., Rana, N., Målqvist, M., Ranneberg, L. J., Subedi, K., & Andersson, O. (2017). Effects of delayed umbilical cord clamping vs early clamping on anemia in infants at 8 and 12 months: a randomized clinical trial. *JAMA Pediatrics, 171*(3), 264–270.

Andersson, O., Hellström-Westas, L., Andersson, D., & Domellöf, M. (2011). Effect of delayed versus early umbilical cord clamping on neonatal outcomes and iron status at 4 months: a randomised controlled trial. *BMJ, 343*, d7157.

Rana, N., Ashish, K. C., Målqvist, M., Subedi, K., & Andersson, O. (2019). Effect of Delayed Cord Clamping of Term Babies on Neurodevelopment at 12 Months: A Randomized Controlled Trial. *Neonatology, 115*(1), 36–42

Andersson, O., Hellström-Westas, L., Andersson, D., & Domellöf, M. (2011). Effect of delayed versus early umbilical cord clamping on neonatal outcomes and iron status at 4 months: a randomised controlled trial. *BMJ, 343*, d7157.

12 Mercer, J. S., Erickson-Owens, D. A., Deoni, S. C., Dean III, D. C., Collins, J., Parker, A. B., … & Padbury, J. F. (2018). Effects of Delayed Cord Clamping on 4-Month Ferritin Levels, Brain Myelin

Content, and Neurodevelopment: A Randomized Controlled Trial. *The Journal of Pediatrics, 203*, 266–272.

13 Mercer, J. S., Erickson-Owens, D. A., Deoni, S. C., Dean III, D. C., Collins, J., Parker, A. B., ... & Padbury, J. F. (2018). Effects of Delayed Cord Clamping on 4-Month Ferritin Levels, Brain Myelin Content, and Neurodevelopment: A Randomized Controlled Trial. *The Journal of Pediatrics, 203*, 266–272.

14 American College of Obstetricians and Gynecologists (2017), Committee Opinion Number 684. Delayed Umbilical Cord Clamping After Birth.

15 Seidler, A. L., Libesman, S., Hunter, K. E., Barba, A., Aberoumand, M., Williams, J. G., ... & Garg, A. (2023). Short, medium, and long deferral of umbilical cord clamping compared with umbilical cord milking and immediate clamping at preterm birth: a systematic review and network meta-analysis with individual participant data. *The Lancet.*

16 Chiruvolu, A., Mallett, L. H., Govande, V. P., Raju, V. N., Hammonds, K., & Katheria, A. C. (2022). Variations in umbilical cord clamping practices in the United States: a national survey of neonatologists. *The Journal of Maternal-Fetal & Neonatal Medicine*, 35(19), 3646-3652.

17 CBR (2019). *Your Guide to Delayed Cord Clamping*. https://www.cordblood.com/how-banking-works/delayed-cord-clamping

18 Janoudi, G., Kelly, S., Yasseen, A., Hamam, H., Moretti, F., & Walker, M. (2015). Factors associated with increased rates of caesarean section in women of advanced maternal age. *Journal of Obstetrics and Gynaecology Canada*, 37(6), 517-526.

Chapter 18. Breastfeeding and the Formula Wars

1 Kramer, M. S., Chalmers, B., Hodnett, E. D., Sevkovskaya, Z., Dzikovich, I., Shapiro, S., ... & Shishko, G. (2001). Promotion of Breastfeeding Intervention Trial (PROBIT): a randomized trial in the Republic of Belarus. *JAMA, 285*(4), 413–420.
Kramer, M. S., Aboud, F., Mironova, E., Vanilovich, I., Platt, R. W., Matush, L., ... & Collet, J. P. (2008). Breastfeeding and child cognitive development: new evidence from a large randomized trial. *Archives of General Psychiatry, 65*(5), 578–584.

2   Evenhouse, E., & Reilly, S. (2005). Improved estimates of the benefits of breastfeeding using sibling comparisons to reduce selection bias. *Health Services Research, 40*(6p1), 1781–1802.

3   Anderson, J. W., Johnstone, B. M., & Remley, D. T. (1999). Breast-feeding and cognitive development: a meta-analysis. *The American Journal of Clinical Nutrition, 70*(4), 525–535.

4   Duijts, L., Jaddoe, V. W., Hofman, A., & Moll, H. A. (2010). Prolonged and exclusive breastfeeding reduces the risk of infectious diseases in infancy. *Pediatrics, peds-2008.*
    Kramer, M. S., Chalmers, B., Hodnett, E. D., Sevkovskaya, Z., Dzikovich, I., Shapiro, S., ... & Shishko, G. (2001). Promotion of Breastfeeding Intervention Trial (PROBIT): a randomized trial in the Republic of Belarus. *JAMA, 285*(4), 413–420.
    Wilson, J. L., & Wilson, B. H. (2018). Is the" breast is best" mantra an oversimplification?. *The Journal of Family Practice, 67*(6), E1–E9.

5   Spiesel, S. Z. (2006). Tales From the Nursery:The health benefits of breast-feeding may not be what you think. *Slate*, March 27, 2006.

6   Van de Perre, P. (2003). Transfer of antibody via mother's milk. *Vaccine, 21*(24), 3374–3376.

7   Simister, N. E. (2003). Placental transport of immunoglobulin G. *Vaccine, 21*(24), 3365–3369.

8   Spiesel, S. Z. (2006). Tales From the Nursery: The health benefits of breast-feeding may not be what you think. *Slate*, March 27, 2006

9   Raissian, K. M., & Su, J. H. (2018). The best of intentions: Prenatal breastfeeding intentions and infant health. *SSM-Population Health, 5*, 86–100.

10 Tuteur, A. (2018). *Mothers who intended to breastfeed had infants with better health outcomes even if they DIDN'T breastfeed!* http://www.skepticalob.com/2018/09/mothers-who-intended-to-breastfeed-had-infants-with-better-health-outcomes-even-if-they-didnt-breastfeed.html

11 Van Odijk, J., Kull, I., Borres, M. P., Brandtzaeg, P., Edberg, U., Hanson, L. Å., ... & Sundell, J. (2003). Breastfeeding and allergic disease: a multidisciplinary review of the literature (1966–2001) on the mode of early feeding in infancy and its impact on later atopic manifestations. *Allergy, 58*(9), 833–843.

12 Lodge, C. J., Tan, D. J., Lau, M. X. Z., Dai, X., Tham, R., Lowe, A. J., ... & Dharmage, S. C. (2015). Breastfeeding and asthma and

allergies: a systematic review and meta-analysis. *Acta Paediatrica, 104*, 38–53.

Van Odijk, J., Kull, I., Borres, M. P., Brandtzaeg, P., Edberg, U., Hanson, L. Å., ... & Sundell, J. (2003). Breastfeeding and allergic disease: a multidisciplinary review of the literature (1966–2001) on the mode of early feeding in infancy and its impact on later atopic manifestations. *Allergy, 58*(9), 833–843.

13 Bezirtzoglou, E., Tsiotsias, A., & Welling, G. W. (2011). Microbiota profile in feces of breast-and formula-fed newborns by using fluorescence in situ hybridization (FISH). *Anaerobe, 17*(6), 478–482.

Mackie, R. I., Sghir, A., & Gaskins, H. R. (1999). Developmental microbial ecology of the neonatal gastrointestinal tract. *The American Journal of Clinical Nutrition, 69*(5), 1035s–1045s.

14 Lodge, C. J., Tan, D. J., Lau, M. X. Z., Dai, X., Tham, R., Lowe, A. J., ... & Dharmage, S. C. (2015). Breastfeeding and asthma and allergies: a systematic review and meta-analysis. *Acta Paediatrica, 104*, 38–53.

15 Arslanoglu, S., Moro, G. E., Schmitt, J., Tandoi, L., Rizzardi, S., & Boehm, G. (2008). Early dietary intervention with a mixture of prebiotic oligosaccharides reduces the incidence of allergic manifestations and infections during the first two years of life. *The Journal of Nutrition, 138*(6), 1091–1095.

Osborn, D. A., & Sinn, J. K. (2013). Prebiotics in infants for prevention of allergy. *Cochrane Database of Systematic Reviews*, (3).

Moro, G., Arslanoglu, S., Stahl, B., Jelinek, J., Wahn, U., & Boehm, G. (2006). A mixture of prebiotic oligosaccharides reduces the incidence of atopic dermatitis during the first six months of age. *Archives of Disease in Childhood, 91*(10), 814–819.

Bruzzese, E., Volpicelli, M., Squeglia, V., Bruzzese, D., Salvini, F., Bisceglia, M., ... & Guarino, A. (2009). A formula containing galacto-and fructo-oligosaccharides prevents intestinal and extra-intestinal infections: an observational study. *Clinical Nutrition, 28*(2), 156–161.

16 Jensen, C. L., Voigt, R. G., Prager, T. C., Zou, Y. L., Fraley, J. K., Rozelle, J. C., ... & Heird, W. C. (2005). Effects of maternal docosahexaenoic acid intake on visual function and neurodevelopment in breastfed term infants. *The American Journal of Clinical Nutrition, 82*(1), 125–132.

Cunnane, S. C., Francescutti, V., Brenna, J. T., & Crawford, M. A. (2000). Breast-fed infants achieve a higher rate of brain and whole body docosahexaenoate accumulation than formula-fed infants not consuming dietary docosahexaenoate. *Lipids, 35*(1), 105–111.

17 Birch, E. E., Garfield, S., Castañeda, Y., Hughbanks-Wheaton, D., Uauy, R., & Hoffman, D. (2007). Visual acuity and cognitive outcomes at 4 years of age in a double-blind, randomized trial of long-chain polyunsaturated fatty acid-supplemented infant formula. *Early Human Development, 83*(5), 279–284.
Qawasmi, A., Landeros-Weisenberger, A., Leckman, J. F., & Bloch, M. H. (2012). Meta-analysis of long-chain polyunsaturated fatty acid supplementation of formula and infant cognition. *Pediatrics, 129*(6), 1141–1149.

18 Timby, N., Domellöf, E., Hernell, O., Lönnerdal, B., & Domellöf, M. (2014). Neurodevelopment, nutrition, and growth until 12 mo of age in infants fed a low-energy, low-protein formula supplemented with bovine milk fat globule membranes: a randomized controlled trial. *The American Journal of Clinical Nutrition, 99*(4), 860–868.
Hernell, O., Domellöf, M., Grip, T., Lönnerdal, B., & Timby, N. (2019). Physiological Effects of Feeding Infants and Young Children Formula Supplemented with Milk Fat Globule Membranes. *In Human Milk: Composition, Clinical Benefits and Future Opportunities* (Vol. 90, pp. 35–42). Karger Publishers.

19 Centers for Disease Control. (2019) *Nationwide Breastfeeding Data & Statistics.* https://www.cdc.gov/breastfeeding/data/facts.html

20 Neifert, M. R. (2001). Prevention of breastfeeding tragedies. *Pediatric Clinics, 48*(2), 273–297.

21 Johns Hopkins Medicine. Breastfeeding and Delayed Milk Production. https://www.hopkinsmedicine.org/health/conditions-and-diseases/breastfeeding-and-delayed-milk-production.

22 *Shared with permission.* del Castillo-Hegyi (2015). https://fedisbest.org/2015/04/letter-to-doctors-and-parents-about-the-dangers-of-insufficient-exclusive-breastfeeding/

23 Seske, L. M., Merhar, S. L., & Haberman, B. E. (2015). Late-onset hypoglycemia in term newborns with poor breastfeeding. *Hospital Pediatrics, 5*(9), 501–504.

24 Flaherman, V. J., Aby, J., Burgos, A. E., Lee, K. A., Cabana, M. D., & Newman, T. B. (2013). Effect of early limited formula on

duration and exclusivity of breastfeeding in at-risk infants: an RCT. *Pediatrics, peds-2012.*

25 Flaherman, V. J., Narayan, N. R., Hartigan-O'Connor, D., Cabana, M. D., McCulloch, C. E., & Paul, I. M. (2018). The effect of early limited formula on breastfeeding, readmission, and intestinal microbiota: a randomized clinical trial. *The Journal of Pediatrics, 196,* 84–90.

26 Tam, E. W., Haeusslein, L. A., Bonifacio, S. L., Glass, H. C., Rogers, E. E., Jeremy, R. J., … & Ferriero, D. M. (2012). Hypoglycemia is associated with increased risk for brain injury and adverse neurodevelopmental outcome in neonates at risk for encephalopathy. *The Journal of Pediatrics, 161*(1), 88–93.

27 Tam, E. W., Haeusslein, L. A., Bonifacio, S. L., Glass, H. C., Rogers, E. E., Jeremy, R. J., … & Ferriero, D. M. (2012). Hypoglycemia is associated with increased risk for brain injury and adverse neurodevelopmental outcome in neonates at risk for encephalopathy. *The Journal of Pediatrics, 161*(1), 88–93.

28 McKinlay, C. J., Alsweiler, J. M., Anstice, N. S., Burakevych, N., Chakraborty, A., Chase, J. G., … & Paudel, N. (2017). Association of neonatal glycemia with neurodevelopmental outcomes at 4.5 years. *JAMA Pediatrics, 171*(10), 972–983.

29 Fed Is Best Foundation (2018) https://fedisbest.org/wp-content/uploads/2018/09/2018-Edition-Feeding-Plan-for-Baby-2.pdf

30 Flaherman, V. J., Cabana, M. D., McCulloch, C. E., & Paul, I. M. Effect of Early Limited Formula on Breastfeeding Duration in the First Year of Life. *JAMA Pediatrics*, 2019; Flaherman, V. J., Narayan, N. R., Hartigan-O'Connor, D., Cabana, M. D., McCulloch, C. E., & Paul, I. M. (2018). The effect of early limited formula on breastfeeding, readmission, and intestinal microbiota: a randomized clinical trial. *The Journal of Pediatrics, 196,* 84–90.

31 Bumrungpert, A., Somboonpanyakul, P., Pavadhgul, P., & Thaninthranon, S. (2018). Effects of fenugreek, ginger, and turmeric supplementation on human milk volume and nutrient content in breastfeeding mothers: A randomized double-blind controlled trial. *Breastfeeding Medicine*, 13(10), 645-650.

32 Huang, S. K., & Chih, M. H. (2020). Increased breastfeeding frequency enhances milk production and infant weight gain:

correlation with the basal maternal prolactin level. Breastfeeding Medicine, 15(10), 639-645.

33 Mitchell, K. B., Johnson, H. M., Rodríguez, J. M., Eglash, A., Scherzinger, C., Widmer, K., ... & Academy of Breastfeeding Medicine. (2022). Academy of Breastfeeding Medicine Clinical Protocol# 36: the mastitis spectrum, revised 2022. *Breastfeeding Medicine*, 17(5), 360-376.

34 Drugs and Lactation Database (LactMed®) [Internet]. Bethesda (MD): National Institute of Child Health and Human Development; 2006-. Ibuprofen. [Updated 2023 Nov 15]. Available from: https://www.ncbi.nlm.nih.gov/books/NBK500986/

35 Douglas, P. (2022). Re-thinking benign inflammation of the lactating breast: classification, prevention, and management. *Women's Health*, 18, 17455057221091349.

36 Korsmo, H. W., Jiang, X., & Caudill, M. A. (2019). Choline: exploring the growing science on its benefits for moms and babies. *Nutrients*, 11(8), 1823.

37 Warstedt, K., Furuhjelm, C., Fälth-Magnusson, K., Fagerås, M., & Duchén, K. (2016). High levels of omega-3 fatty acids in milk from omega-3 fatty acid-supplemented mothers are related to less immunoglobulin E-associated disease in infancy. *Acta Paediatrica*, 105(11), 1337-1347.

Chapter 19. Choosing a Formula

1 Tolia, V., Lin, C. H., & Kuhns, L. R. (1992). Gastric emptying using three different formulas in infants with gastroesophageal reflux. *Journal of Pediatric Gastroenterology and Nutrition, 15*(3), 297–301.

2

3 Kanabar, D., Randhawa, M., & Clayton, P. (2001). Improvement of symptoms in infant colic following reduction of lactose load with lactase. *Journal of Human Nutrition and Dietetics, 14*(5), 359–363.
Ståhlberg, M. R., & Savilahti, E. (1986). Infantile colic and feeding. *Archives of Disease in Childhood, 61*(12), 1232–1233.
Miller JJ, McVeagh P, Fleet GH, et al. Effect of yeast lactase enzyme on "colic" in infants fed human milk. *J Pediatr 1990; 117* (2 Pt 1), 261–263

4   Francavilla, R., Calasso, M., Calace, L., Siragusa, S., Ndagijimana,
    M., Vernocchi, P., ... & Indrio, F. (2012). Effect of lactose on gut
    microbiota and metabolome of infants with cow's milk allergy.
    Pediatric Allergy and Immunology, 23(5), 420–427.
5   Bosheva, M., Tokodi, I., Krasnow, A., Pedersen, H. K.,
    Lukjancenko, O., Eklund, A. C., ... & HMO Study Investigator
    Consortium. (2022). Infant formula with a specific blend of
    five human milk oligosaccharides drives the gut microbiota
    development and improves gut maturation markers: A
    randomized controlled trial. *Frontiers in Nutrition, 9*, 920362.
    Holst, A. Q., Myers, P., Rodríguez-García, P., Hermes, G. D.,
    Melsaether, C., Baker, A., ... & Parschat, K. (2023). Infant Formula
    Supplemented with Five Human Milk Oligosaccharides Shifts
    the Fecal Microbiome of Formula-Fed Infants Closer to That of
    Breastfed Infants. *Nutrients, 15*(14), 3087.
6   Ben, X. M., Li, J., Feng, Z. T., Shi, S. Y., Lu, Y. D., Chen, R., & Zhou,
    X. Y. (2008). Low level of galacto-oligosaccharide in infant formula
    stimulates growth of intestinal Bifidobacteria and Lactobacilli.
    World Journal of Gastroenterology: WJG, 14(42), 6564.
    Matsuki, T., Tajima, S., Hara, T., Yahagi, K., Ogawa, E., &
    Kodama, H. (2016). Infant formula with galacto-oligosaccharides
    (OM55N) stimulates the growth of indigenous bifidobacteria in
    healthy term infants. *Beneficial Microbes, 7*(4), 453–461.
    Cai, J. W., Lu, Y. D., & Ben, X. M. (2008). Effects of infant formula
    containing galacto-oligosaccharides on the intestinal microflora
    in infants. *Zhongguo dang dai er ke za zhi= Chinese Journal of
    Contemporary Pediatrics, 10*(5), 629–632.
    Rinne, M. M., Gueimonde, M., Kalliomäki, M., Hoppu, U.,
    Salminen, S. J., & Isolauri, E. (2005). Similar bifidogenic effects of
    prebiotic-supplemented partially hydrolyzed infant formula and
    breastfeeding on infant gut microbiota. *FEMS Immunology &
    Medical Microbiology, 43*(1), 59–65.
7   Cool, R., & Vandenplas, Y. (2023). The Link between Different
    Types of Prebiotics in Infant Formula and Infection Rates: A
    Review. *Nutrients, 15*(8), 1942.
    Arslanoglu, S., Moro, G. E., Schmitt, J., Tandoi, L., Rizzardi, S.,
    & Boehm, G. (2008). Early dietary intervention with a mixture
    of prebiotic oligosaccharides reduces the incidence of allergic

manifestations and infections during the first two years of life. *The Journal of Nutrition, 138*(6), 1091–1095.

Osborn, D. A., & Sinn, J. K. (2013). Prebiotics in infants for prevention of allergy. *Cochrane Database of Systematic Reviews*, (3).

Moro, G., Arslanoglu, S., Stahl, B., Jelinek, J., Wahn, U., & Boehm, G. (2006). A mixture of prebiotic oligosaccharides reduces the incidence of atopic dermatitis during the first six months of age. *Archives of Disease in Childhood, 91*(10), 814–819.

Bruzzese, E., Volpicelli, M., Squeglia, V., Bruzzese, D., Salvini, F., Bisceglia, M., ... & Guarino, A. (2009). A formula containing galacto-and fructo-oligosaccharides prevents intestinal and extra-intestinal infections: an observational study. *Clinical Nutrition, 28*(2), 156–161.

8   Cool, R., & Vandenplas, Y. (2023). The Link between Different Types of Prebiotics in Infant Formula and Infection Rates: A Review. *Nutrients*, 15(8), 1942.

Arslanoglu, S., Moro, G. E., Schmitt, J., Tandoi, L., Rizzardi, S., & Boehm, G. (2008). Early dietary intervention with a mixture of prebiotic oligosaccharides reduces the incidence of allergic manifestations and infections during the first two years of life. *The Journal of Nutrition, 138*(6), 1091–1095.

Osborn, D. A., & Sinn, J. K. (2013). Prebiotics in infants for prevention of allergy. *Cochrane Database of Systematic Reviews*, (3).

Moro, G., Arslanoglu, S., Stahl, B., Jelinek, J., Wahn, U., & Boehm, G. (2006). A mixture of prebiotic oligosaccharides reduces the incidence of atopic dermatitis during the first six months of age. *Archives of Disease in Childhood, 91*(10), 814–819.

Bruzzese, E., Volpicelli, M., Squeglia, V., Bruzzese, D., Salvini, F., Bisceglia, M., ... & Guarino, A. (2009). A formula containing galacto-and fructo-oligosaccharides prevents intestinal and extra-intestinal infections: an observational study. *Clinical Nutrition, 28*(2), 156–161.

9   Ivakhnenko, O. S., & Nyankovskyy, S. L. (2013). Effect of the specific infant formula mixture of oligosaccharides on local immunity and development of allergic and infectious disease in young children: randomized study. *Pediatria Polska, 88*(5), 398–404.

10 Cuello-Garcia, C. A., Fiocchi, A., Pawankar, R., Yepes-Nuñez, J. J., Morgano, G. P., Zhang, Y., ... & Beyer, K. (2016). World allergy organization-McMaster University guidelines for allergic disease

prevention (GLAD-P): Prebiotics. *World Allergy Organization Journal*, 9(1), 10.

11 Bosheva, M., Tokodi, I., Krasnow, A., Pedersen, H. K., Lukjancenko, O., Eklund, A. C., ... & HMO Study Investigator Consortium. (2022). Infant formula with a specific blend of five human milk oligosaccharides drives the gut microbiota development and improves gut maturation markers: A randomized controlled trial. *Frontiers in Nutrition*, 9, 920362.

12 Lenehan, S. M., Boylan, G. B., Livingstone, V., Fogarty, L., Twomey, D. M., Nikolovski, J., ... & Murray, D. M. (2020). The impact of short-term predominate breastfeeding on cognitive outcome at 5 years. *Acta Paediatrica*, 109(5), 982-988.

13 Schipper, L., Bartke, N., Marintcheva-Petrova, M., Schoen, S., Vandenplas, Y., & Hokken-Koelega, A. C. (2023). Infant formula containing large, milk phospholipid-coated lipid droplets and dairy lipids affects cognitive performance at school age. *Frontiers in Nutrition*, 10.

Nieto-Ruiz, A., García-Santos, J. A., Verdejo-Román, J., Diéguez, E., Sepúlveda-Valbuena, N., Herrmann, F., ... & Campoy, C. (2022). Infant formula supplemented with milk fat globule membrane, long-chain polyunsaturated fatty acids, and synbiotics is associated with neurocognitive function and brain structure of healthy children aged 6 years: the COGNIS study. *Frontiers in Nutrition*, 9, 820224.

Xia, Y., Jiang, B., Zhou, L., Ma, J., Yang, L., Wang, F., ... & Wang, B. (2021). Neurodevelopmental outcomes of healthy Chinese term infants fed infant formula enriched in bovine milk fat globule membrane for 12 months-A randomized controlled trial. *Asia Pacific Journal of Clinical Nutrition*, 30(3), 401-414.

Timby, N., Domellöf, E., Hernell, O., Lönnerdal, B., & Domellöf, M. (2014). Neurodevelopment, nutrition, and growth until 12 mo of age in infants fed a low-energy, low-protein formula supplemented with bovine milk fat globule membranes: a randomized controlled trial. *The American Journal of Clinical Nutrition*, 99(4), 860–868.

14 Timby, N., Adamsson, M., Domellöf, E., Grip, T., Hernell, O., Lönnerdal, B., & Domellöf, M. (2021). Neurodevelopment and growth until 6.5 years of infants who consumed a low-energy, low-protein formula supplemented with bovine milk fat globule

membranes: a randomized controlled trial. *The American Journal of Clinical Nutrition*, 113(3), 586-592.

15 Bhinder, G., Allaire, J. M., Garcia, C., Lau, J. T., Chan, J. M., Ryz, N. R., ... & Berkmann, J. C. (2017). Milk fat globule membrane supplementation in formula modulates the neonatal gut microbiome and normalizes intestinal development. *Scientific Reports, 7*, 45274

16 Brink, L. R., Herren, A. W., McMillen, S., Fraser, K., Agnew, M., Roy, N., & Lönnerdal, B. (2020). Omics analysis reveals variations among commercial sources of bovine milk fat globule membrane. *Journal of Dairy Science*, 103(4), 3002-3016.

17 Ochoa, T. J., Chea-Woo, E., Baiocchi, N., Pecho, I., Campos, M., Prada, A., ... & Cleary, T. G. (2013). Randomized double-blind controlled trial of bovine lactoferrin for prevention of diarrhea in children. *The Journal of Pediatrics, 162*(2), 349–356.

Pammi, M., & Suresh, G. (2017). Enteral lactoferrin supplementation for prevention of sepsis and necrotizing enterocolitis in preterm infants. *Cochrane Database of Systematic Reviews*, (6).

Donovan, S. M. (2016). The role of lactoferrin in gastrointestinal and immune development and function: a preclinical perspective. *The Journal of Pediatrics, 173*, S16–S28.

Pammi, M., & Abrams, S. A. (2015). Oral lactoferrin for the prevention of sepsis and necrotizing enterocolitis in preterm infants. *Cochrane Database of Systematic Reviews*, (2).

18 Melgar, M. J., Santaeufemia, M., & García, M. A. (2010). Organophosphorus pesticide residues in raw milk and infant formulas from Spanish northwest. *Journal of Environmental Science and Health Part B, 45*(7), 595–600.

19 Cressey, P. J., & Vannoort, R. W. (2003). Pesticide content of infant formulae and weaning foods available in New Zealand. *Food Additives & Contaminants, 20*(1), 57–64.

Gelardi, R. C., & Mountford, M. K. (1993). Infant formulas: evidence of the absence of pesticide residues. *Regulatory Toxicology and Pharmacology, 17*(2), 181–192.

Chen, X., Panuwet, P., Hunter, R. E., Riederer, A. M., Bernoudy, G. C., Barr, D. B., & Ryan, P. B. (2014). Method for the quantification of current use and persistent pesticides in cow milk, human milk and baby formula using gas chromatography tandem mass spectrometry. *Journal of Chromatography B, 970*, 121–130.

20 Pico, Y., Viana, E., Font, G., & Manes, J. (1995). Determination of organochlorine pesticide content in human milk and infant formulas using solid phase extraction and capillary gas chromatography. *Journal of Agricultural and Food Chemistry, 43*(6), 1610–1615.

Chapter 20. Newborn Probiotics and Vitamin D

1 Kennedy, K. M., de Goffau, M. C., Perez-Muñoz, M. E., Arrieta, M. C., Bäckhed, F., Bork, P., ... & Walter, J. (2023). Questioning the fetal microbiome illustrates pitfalls of low-biomass microbial studies. *Nature, 613*(7945), 639-649.

2 Bager, P., Wohlfahrt, J., & Westergaard, T. (2008). Caesarean delivery and risk of atopy and allergic disesase: meta-analyses. *Clinical & Experimental Allergy, 38*(4), 634-642.

Azad, M. B., Konya, T., Guttman, D. S., Field, C. J., Sears, M. R., HayGlass, K. T., ... & Scott, J. A. (2015). Infant gut microbiota and food sensitization: associations in the first year of life. *Clinical & Experimental Allergy, 45*(3), 632–643.

Metsälä, J., Lundqvist, A., Virta, L. J., Kaila, M., Gissler, M., & Virtanen, S. M. (2013). Mother's and offspring's use of antibiotics and infant allergy to cow's milk. *Epidemiology*, 303–309.

Sjögren, Y. M., Jenmalm, M. C., Böttcher, M. F., Björkstén, B., & Sverremark-Ekström, E. (2009). Altered early infant gut microbiota in children developing allergy up to 5 years of age. *Clinical & Experimental Allergy, 39*(4), 518–526.

Abrahamsson, T. R., Jakobsson, H. E., Andersson, A. F., Björkstén, B., Engstrand, L., & Jenmalm, M. C. (2012). Low diversity of the gut microbiota in infants with atopic eczema. *Journal of Allergy and Clinical Immunology, 129*(2), 434–440.

Penders, J., Gerhold, K., Stobberingh, E. E., Thijs, C., Zimmermann, K., Lau, S., & Hamelmann, E. (2013). Establishment of the intestinal microbiota and its role for atopic dermatitis in early childhood. *Journal of Allergy and Clinical Immunology, 132*(3), 601–607.

Guaraldi, F., & Salvatori, G. (2012). Effect of breast and formula feeding on gut microbiota shaping in newborns. *Frontiers in Cellular and Infection Microbiology, 2*, 94.

3 Casaburi, G., Duar, R. M., Brown, H., Mitchell, R. D., Kazi, S., Chew, S., ... & Freeman, S. L. (2021). Metagenomic insights of

the infant microbiome community structure and function across multiple sites in the United States. *Scientific Reports*, 11(1), 1472.

4 Underwood, M. A., German, J. B., Lebrilla, C. B., & Mills, D. A. (2015). Bifidobacterium longum subspecies infantis: champion colonizer of the infant gut. *Pediatric Research, 77*(1–2), 229.

5 Batta, V. K., Rao, S. C., & Patole, S. K. (2023). Bifidobacterium infantis as a probiotic in preterm infants: a systematic review and meta-analysis. *Pediatric Research*, 94(6), 1887-1905.

6 Underwood, M. A., German, J. B., Lebrilla, C. B., & Mills, D. A. (2015). Bifidobacterium longum subspecies infantis: champion colonizer of the infant gut. *Pediatric Research, 77*(1–2), 229.
Bin-Nun, A., Bromiker, R., Wilschanski, M., Kaplan, M., Rudensky, B., Caplan, M., & Hammerman, C. (2005). Oral probiotics prevent necrotizing enterocolitis in very low birth weight neonates. *The Journal of Pediatrics, 147*(2), 192–196.
Lin, H. C., Su, B. H., Chen, A. C., Lin, T. W., Tsai, C. H., Yeh, T. F., & Oh, W. (2005). Oral probiotics reduce the incidence and severity of necrotizing enterocolitis in very low birth weight infants. *Pediatrics, 115*(1), 1–4.
Kanic, Z., Turk, D. M., Burja, S., Kanic, V., & Dinevski, D. (2015). Influence of a combination of probiotics on bacterial infections in very low birthweight newborns. *Wiener Klinische Wochenschrift, 127*(5), 210–215.
Dermyshi, E., Wang, Y., Yan, C., Hong, W., Qiu, G., Gong, X., & Zhang, T. (2017). The "golden age" of probiotics: a systematic review and meta-analysis of randomized and observational studies in preterm infants. *Neonatology, 112*(1), 9–23.

7 Henrick, B. M., Hutton, A. A., Palumbo, M. C., Casaburi, G., Mitchell, R. D., Underwood, M. A., … & Frese, S. A. (2018). Elevated fecal pH indicates a profound change in the breastfed infant gut microbiome due to reduction of Bifidobacterium over the past century. *mSphere, 3*(2), e00041–18.

8 Henrick, B. M., Hutton, A. A., Palumbo, M. C., Casaburi, G., Mitchell, R. D., Underwood, M. A., … & Frese, S. A. (2018). Elevated fecal pH indicates a profound change in the breastfed infant gut microbiome due to reduction of Bifidobacterium over the past century. *mSphere, 3*(2), e00041–18.

9 Seppo, A. E., Bu, K., Jumabaeva, M., Thakar, J., Choudhury, R. A., Yonemitsu, C., … & Järvinen, K. M. (2021). Infant gut

microbiome is enriched with Bifidobacterium longum ssp. infantis in Old Order Mennonites with traditional farming lifestyle. *Allergy, 76*(11), 3489-3503.

10 Henrick, B. M., Chew, S., Prambs, J., Brown, H. K., Underwood, M., Smilowitz, J. T., ... & German, B. (2021). B. infantis EVC001 Colonization in Breastfed Infants Modulates Cytokine Profile Linked to Autoimmune and Allergic Diseases. *Pediatrics, 147*(3_ MeetingAbstract), 684-685.

Frese, S. A., Hutton, A. A., Contreras, L. N., Shaw, C. A., Palumbo, M. C., Casaburi, G., ... & Freeman, S. L. (2017). Persistence of Supplemented Bifidobacterium longum subsp. infantis EVC001 in Breastfed Infants. *mSphere, 2*(6), e00501-17.

Casaburi, G., & Frese, S. A. (2018). Colonization of breastfed infants by Bifidobacterium longum subsp. infantis EVC001 reduces virulence gene abundance. *Human Microbiome Journal, 9*, 7-10.

Karav, S., Casaburi, G., & Frese, S. A. (2018). Reduced colonic mucin degradation in breastfed infants colonized by Bifidobacterium longum subsp. infantis EVC001. *FEBS Open Bio, 8*(10), 1649-1657.

Chen, L., Ni, Y., Wu, X., & Chen, G. (2022). Probiotics for the prevention of atopic dermatitis in infants from different geographic regions: a systematic review and Meta-analysis. *Journal of Dermatological Treatment, 33*(7), 2931-2939.

11 Korpela, K., Salonen, A., Vepsäläinen, O., Suomalainen, M., Kolmeder, C., Varjosalo, M., ... & de Vos, W. M. (2018). Probiotic supplementation restores normal microbiota composition and function in antibiotic-treated and in caesarean-born infants. *Microbiome, 6*(1), 182.

Underwood, M. A., German, J. B., Lebrilla, C. B., & Mills, D. A. (2015). Bifidobacterium longum subspecies infantis: champion colonizer of the infant gut. *Pediatric Research, 77*(1-2), 229.

Ganguli, K., Collado, M. C., Rautava, J., Lu, L., Satokari, R., von Ossowski, I., ... & Salminen, S. (2015). Lactobacillus rhamnosus GG and its SpaC pilus adhesin modulate inflammatory responsiveness and TLR-related gene expression in the fetal human gut. *Pediatric Research, 77*(4), 528.

Capurso, L. (2019). Thirty Years of Lactobacillus rhamnosus GG: A Review. *Journal of Clinical Gastroenterology, 53*, S1–S41.

De Andrés, J., Manzano, S., García, C., Rodríguez, J. M., Espinosa-Martos, I., & Jiménez, E. (2018). Modulatory effect of three probiotic strains on infants' gut microbial composition and immunological parameters on a placebo-controlled, double-blind, randomised study. *Beneficial Microbes, 9*(4), 573–584.

12 Ang, J. L., Athalye-Jape, G., Rao, S., Bulsara, M., & Patole, S. (2023). Limosilactobacillus reuteri DSM 17938 as a probiotic in preterm infants: An updated systematic review with meta-analysis and trial sequential analysis. *Journal of Parenteral and Enteral Nutrition*, 47(8), 963-981.

13 Dinleyici, E. C., Dalgic, N., Guven, S., Metin, O., Yasa, O., Kurugol, Z., ... & Vandenplas, Y. (2015). Lactobacillus reuteri DSM 17938 shortens acute infectious diarrhea in a pediatric outpatient setting. *Jornal de pediatria*, 91, 392-396.

14 Banakar, M., Pourhajibagher, M., Etemad-Moghadam, S., Mehran, M., Yazdi, M. H., Haghgoo, R., ... & Frankenberger, R. (2023). Antimicrobial Effects of Postbiotic Mediators Derived from Lactobacillus rhamnosus GG and Lactobacillus reuteri on Streptococcus mutans. *Frontiers in Bioscience-Landmark*, 28(5), 88.
Srinivasan, R., Kesavelu, D., Veligandla, K. C., Muni, S. K., & Mehta, S. C. (2018). Lactobacillus reuteri DSM 17938: Review of evidence in functional gastrointestinal disorders. *Pediatr. Ther*, 8(350), 2161-0665.

15 Rhoads, J. M., Collins, J., Fatheree, N. Y., Hashmi, S. S., Taylor, C. M., Luo, M., ... & Liu, Y. (2018). Infant colic represents gut inflammation and dysbiosis. *The Journal of Pediatrics, 203*, 55–61.

16 Vaz, S. R., Tofoli, M. H., Avelino, M. A. G., & da Costa, P. S. S. (2024). Probiotics for infantile colic: Is there evidence beyond doubt? A meta-analysis and systematic review. *Acta Paediatrica*, 113(2), 170-182.
Rhoads, J. M. (2018). Probiotic Lactobacillus reuteri effective in treating infantile colic and is associated with inflammatory marker reduction. *The Journal of Pediatrics, 196*, 324–327.
Skonieczna-Żydecka, K., Janda, K., Kaczmarczyk, M., Marlicz, W., Łoniewski, I., & Łoniewska, B. (2020). The effect of probiotics on symptoms, gut microbiota and inflammatory markers in infantile colic: a systematic review, meta-analysis and meta-regression of randomized controlled trials. *Journal of Clinical Medicine*, 9(4), 999.

17 Savino, F., Garro, M., Montanari, P., Galliano, I., & Bergallo, M. (2018). Crying time and RORγ/FOXP3 expression in Lactobacillus reuteri DSM17938-treated infants with colic: a randomized trial. *The Journal of Pediatrics, 192*, 171–177.

18 Henrick, B. M., Chew, S., Casaburi, G., Brown, H. K., Frese, S. A., Zhou, Y., … & Smilowitz, J. T. (2019). Colonization by B. infantis EVC001 modulates enteric inflammation in exclusively breastfed infants. *Pediatric Research, 86*(6), 749-757.
    Pärtty, A., Kalliomäki, M., Endo, A., Salminen, S., & Isolauri, E. (2012). Compositional development of Bifidobacterium and Lactobacillus microbiota is linked with crying and fussing in early infancy. *PloS One, 7*(3), e32495.

19 Indrio, F., Di Mauro, A., Riezzo, G., Civardi, E., Intini, C., Corvaglia, L., … & Francavilla, R. (2014). Prophylactic use of a probiotic in the prevention of colic, regurgitation, and functional constipation: a randomized clinical trial. *JAMA Pediatrics, 168*(3), 228-233.

20 Indrio, F., Riezzo, G., Giordano, P., Ficarella, M., Miolla, M. P., Martini, S., … & Francavilla, R. (2017). Effect of a partially hydrolysed whey infant formula supplemented with starch and Lactobacillus reuteri DSM 17938 on regurgitation and gastric motility. *Nutrients, 9*(11), 1181.

21 Mitre, E., Susi, A., Kropp, L. E., Schwartz, D. J., Gorman, G. H., & Nylund, C. M. (2018). Association between use of acid-suppressive medications and antibiotics during infancy and allergic diseases in early childhood. *JAMA Pediatrics, 172*(6), e180315–e180315.

22 Weizman, Z. V. I., Alkrinawi, S., Goldfarb, D. A. N., & Bitran, C. (1993). Efficacy of herbal tea preparation in infantile colic. *The Journal of Pediatrics, 122*(4), 650–652.

23 Yamamoto-Hanada, K., Yang, L., Narita, M., Saito, H., & Ohya, Y. (2017). Influence of antibiotic use in early childhood on asthma and allergic diseases at age 5. *Annals of Allergy, Asthma & Immunology, 119*(1), 54-58.
    Hoskin-Parr, L., Teyhan, A., Blocker, A., & Henderson, A. J. W. (2013). Antibiotic exposure in the first two years of life and development of asthma and other allergic diseases by 7.5 yr: a dose-dependent relationship. *Pediatric Allergy and Immunology, 24*(8), 762-771.

Droste, J. H. J., Wieringa, M. H., Weyler, J. J., Nelen, V. J., Vermeire, P. A., & Van Bever, H. P. (2000). Does the use of antibiotics in early childhood increase the risk of asthma and allergic disease?. *Clinical & Experimental Allergy, 30*(11), 1548–1553.

Kozyrskyj, A. L., Ernst, P., & Becker, A. B. (2007). Increased risk of childhood asthma from antibiotic use in early life. *Chest, 131*(6), 1753–1759.

Kronman, M. P., Zaoutis, T. E., Haynes, K., Feng, R., & Coffin, S. E. (2012). Antibiotic exposure and IBD development among children: a population-based cohort study. *Pediatrics, 130*(4), e794.

Kummeling, I., Stelma, F. F., Dagnelie, P. C., Snijders, B. E., Penders, J., Huber, M., ... & Thijs, C. (2007). Early life exposure to antibiotics and the subsequent development of eczema, wheeze, and allergic sensitization in the first 2 years of life: the KOALA Birth Cohort Study. *Pediatrics*, 119(1), e225-e231.

24 Engelbrektson, A., Korzenik, J. R., Pittler, A., Sanders, M. E., Klaenhammer, T. R., Leyer, G., & Kitts, C. L. (2009). Probiotics to minimize the disruption of faecal microbiota in healthy subjects undergoing antibiotic therapy. *Journal of Medical Microbiology, 58*(5), 663–670.

25 Cremonini, F., Di Caro, S., Nista, E. C., Bartolozzi, F., Capelli, G. Gasbarrini, G., & Gasbarrini, A.(2002). Meta-analysis: the effect of probiotic administration on antibiotic-associated diarrhoea. *Alimentary Pharmacology & Therapeutics, 16*(8), 1461–1467.

Szajewska, H., Canani, R. B., Guarino, A., Hojsak, I., Indrio, F., Kolacek, S., ... & Weizman, Z. (2016). Probiotics for the prevention of antibiotic-associated diarrhea in children. *Journal of Pediatric Gastroenterology and Nutrition, 62*(3), 495–506.

26 Kabbani, T. A., Pallav, K., Dowd, S. E., Villafuerte-Galvez, J., Vanga, R. R., Castillo, N. E., ... & Kelly, C. P. (2017). Prospective randomized controlled study on the effects of Saccharomyces boulardii CNCM I-745 and amoxicillin-clavulanate or the combination on the gut microbiota of healthy volunteers. *Gut Microbes, 8*(1), 17–32.

Korpela, K., Salonen, A., Virta, L. J., Kumpu, M., Kekkonen, R. A., & De Vos, W. M. (2016). Lactobacillus rhamnosus GG intake modifies preschool children's intestinal microbiota, alleviates penicillin-associated changes, and reduces antibiotic use. *PloS One, 11*(4), e0154012.

Szajewska, H., & Kołodziej, M. (2015). Systematic review with meta-analysis: Lactobacillus rhamnosus GG in the prevention of antibiotic-associated diarrhoea in children and adults. *Alimentary Pharmacology & Therapeutics, 42*(10), 1149–1157.

27 Collignon, A., Sandre, C., & Barc, M. C. (2010). Saccharomyces boulardii modulates dendritic cell properties and intestinal microbiota disruption after antibiotic treatment. *Gastroentérologie Clinique et Biologique, 34,* S71–S78.

Bruzzese, E., Callegari, M. L., Raia, V., Viscovo, S., Scotto, R., Ferrari, S., ... & Guarino, A. (2014). Disrupted intestinal microbiota and intestinal inflammation in children with cystic fibrosis and its restoration with Lactobacillus GG: a randomised clinical trial. *PLoS One, 9*(2), e87796.

28 Demirel, G., Celik, I. H., Erdeve, O., Saygan, S., Dilmen, U., & Canpolat, F. E. (2013). Prophylactic Saccharomyces boulardii versus nystatin for the prevention of fungal colonization and invasive fungal infection in premature infants. *European Journal of Pediatrics, 172*(10), 1321–1326.

Demirel, G., Erdeve, O., Celik, I. H., & Dilmen, U. (2013). Saccharomyces boulardii for prevention of necrotizing enterocolitis in preterm infants: a randomized, controlled study. *Acta Paediatrica, 102*(12), e560–e565.

Xu, L., Wang, Y., Wang, Y., Fu, J., Sun, M., Mao, Z., & Vandenplas, Y. (2016). A double-blinded randomized trial on growth and feeding tolerance with Saccharomyces boulardii CNCM I-745 in formula-fed preterm infants. *Jornal de Pediatria (Versão em Português), 92*(3), 296–301.

29 Urashima, M., Segawa, T., Okazaki, M., Kurihara, M., Wada, Y., & Ida, H. (2010). Randomized trial of vitamin D supplementation to prevent seasonal influenza A in schoolchildren. *The American journal of Clinical Nutrition, 91*(5), 1255–1260.

30 Pawley, N., & Bishop, N. J. (2004). Prenatal and infant predictors of bone health: the influence of vitamin D. *The American Journal of Clinical Nutrition, 80*(6), 1748S-1751S.

31 Zipitis, C. S., & Akobeng, A. K. (2008). Vitamin D supplementation in early childhood and risk of type 1 diabetes: a systematic review and meta-analysis. *Archives of Disease in Childhood, 93*(6), 512–517.

Schmidt, R. J., Hansen, R. L., Hartiala, J., Allayee, H., Sconberg, J. L., Schmidt, L. C., … & Tassone, F. (2015). Selected vitamin D metabolic gene variants and risk for autism spectrum disorder in the CHARGE Study. *Early Human Development, 91*(8), 483–489.

Coşkun, S., Şimşek, Ş., Camkurt, M. A., Çim, A., & Çelik, S. B. (2016). Association of polymorphisms in the vitamin D receptor gene and serum 25-hydroxyvitamin D levels in children with autism spectrum disorder. *Gene, 588*(2), 109–114.

Cannell, J. J., & Grant, W. B. (2013). What is the role of vitamin D in autism?. *Dermato-Endocrinology, 5*(1), 199–204.

Kočovská, E., Andorsdóttir, G., Weihe, P., Halling, J., Fernell, E., Stóra, T., … & Bourgeron, T. (2014). Vitamin D in the general population of young adults with autism in the Faroe Islands. *Journal of Autism and Developmental Disorders, 44*(12), 2996–3005.

Stubbs, G., Henley, K., & Green, J. (2016). Autism: will vitamin D supplementation during pregnancy and early childhood reduce the recurrence rate of autism in newborn siblings? *Medical Hypotheses, 88*, 74–78.

32 Gordon, C. M., Feldman, H. A., Sinclair, L., Williams, A. L., Kleinman, P. K., Perez-Rossello, J., & Cox, J. E. (2008). Prevalence of vitamin D deficiency among healthy infants and toddlers. *Archives of Pediatrics & Adolescent Medicine, 162*(6), 505-512.

33 Perrine, C. G., Sharma, A. J., Jefferds, M. E. D., Serdula, M. K., & Scanlon, K. S. (2010). Adherence to vitamin D recommendations among US infants. *Pediatrics, 125*(4), 627.

34 American Academy of Pediatrics. (2010). *Vitamin D Supplementation for Infants.* https://www.aap.org/en-us/about-the-aap/aap-press-room/pages/Vitamin-D-Supplementation-for-Infants.aspx

35 O'Callaghan, K. M., Taghivand, M., Zuchniak, A., Onoyovwi, A., Korsiak, J., Leung, M., & Roth, D. E. (2020). Vitamin D in breastfed infants: systematic review of alternatives to daily supplementation. *Advances in Nutrition*, 11(1), 144-159.

Hollis, B. W., Wagner, C. L., Howard, C. R., Ebeling, M., Shary, J. R., Smith, P. G., … & Hulsey, T. C. (2015). Maternal versus infant vitamin D supplementation during lactation: a randomized controlled trial. *Pediatrics*, 136(4), 625-634.

Index

Made in the USA
Las Vegas, NV
03 November 2024

10527870R00204